Beating
Osteoporosis
Naturally
Easily
Sensibly

Beating
Osteoporosis
Naturally
Easily
Sensibly

Everything you need to know
About your bones and osteoporosis
Understanding—Prevention—Cure

By Robert Pirello
with Bernardo Merizalde, MD

"Diet for Healthy Bones" and over 150 "Recipes for Healthy Bones"
by Christina Pirello

Author of: *Cooking The Whole Foods Way*

And Emmy Award-winning host of Public Television's & CN8 The Comcast
Network's 'Christina Cooks'

Library of Congress Control Number:		2006910183
ISBN 10 :	Hardcover	1-4257-4389-7
	Softcover	1-4257-4388-9
ISBN 13 :	Hardcover	978-1-4257-4389-5
	Softcover	978-1-4257-4388-8

This book was printed in the United States of America.

To order additional copies of this book, contact:
Xlibris Corporation
1-888-795-4274
www.Xlibris.com
Orders@Xlibris.com
37201

Contents

Part Three - The Diet Connection

To the two people who have motivated and inspired my adult life more than anyone else.

For my wife
Christina Pirello
You make me laugh, smile and you inspire me, (and many others), unconditionally.

And for
Don Young
My running partner since 1983, and who at 60 plus can still run ten marathons a year.

.

A Message to the Reader

The ideas, procedures, and suggestions contained in this book are not intended to treat or diagnosis osteoporosis, nor are they a substitute for medical treatment by a physician. If you have osteoporosis, you are at constant risk of fracture. Do not stop taking any prescribed medications unless advised to do so by your physician, and do not take on an exercise program without your doctor's knowledge and professional supervision. The reader should always consult a physician in matters relating to health.

Acknowledgements

Books don't just happen as a result of one person sitting down at a computer and writing. They are a result of years of living and being. They are made up of the experiences of a lifetime; and they are inspired by the lives of many.

I owe a dept of gratitude to my co-authors, my wonderful wife and partner, Christina, and to my good friend Bernardo Merizalde, M.D. Their commitment and contribution to this work gave it life, made it possible, and are forever greatly appreciated.

I will always be deeply grateful to my many running buddies who both encouraged and inspired me to remain focused on regaining my health and strength, reassuring me that I had it in me to fully recover and run another marathon.

To Jeff and all of the physical therapists at Excel Physical Therapy, who pushed me beyond my limits at each and every physical therapy session.

To Dr. Ray Moyer at Temple University Center for Sports Medicine and Science . . . I have seen this fine doctor over the years for many sports related injuries.

To all of the people who struggle with osteoporosis that I have encountered since my diagnosis in 1998. You have been my greatest source of inspiration. This book is for you.

Preface

I met Christina and Robert a number of years ago when they became interested in my practice of alternative medicine and homeopathy. When I met Robert, he was suffering from severe osteoporosis. He shares with us his riveting story, and it is an inspiring and motivating one.

With his strength and desire to transform his condition he engaged in searching for answers and approaches that would benefit him. Robert took on the quest of learning everything there was to be known about osteoporosis and share his knowledge and experience with the public. Since then, we have collaborated in helping many individuals suffering from this potentially limiting disorder. This book is the compilation of our findings, literature reviews, continuing education and from our work.

As you will find, osteoporosis is not a clear cut condition, but is the result of various factors, genetic and environmental, that start interacting from early life, especially from adolescence. It is important to adopt an attitude of prevention by educating our youth about the various controllable risk factors to avoid osteoporosis.

Furthermore, the factors that predispose to osteoporosis also participate in the manifestation of other disorders like cardiovascular disorders, including heart attacks and stroke, cancer and probably other degenerative disorders like arthritis and dementia.

Recently, the United States Department of Agriculture revised the food pyramid to reflect scientific findings and to recommend the consumption of vegetables while decreasing the content of animal fats and protein. Sadly, these findings of the impact of diet on health have been available for at least twenty years and just now are they making their way into the conventional literature. Therefore, it is important for people to take an active role in their healthcare and not wait for the official establishment to stamp their approval on sensible and safe approaches that have reasonable research published in independent magazines.

It is hard to change behavior patterns that predispose us to negative consequences to our health. To eat properly and avoid junk food, to be physically active and not be a couch potato requires insight, motivation and will. To achieve change and develop ourselves into the best we can be, can be an emotionally gratifying experience. We encourage you to take the steps in this book with interest and curiosity and see how far you can go. You will find in the bibliography various references that will expand your knowledge, strategies and techniques that will help you to address more specifically, and in detail, particular blocks and challenges encountered on the way to healing. You will heal more than your bones.

We still don't have a definitive blueprint to the human being. Science is still looking for and finding ever more complex biochemical reactions in every organ system. We have included as much as is readily available to us, to this date on the subject of osteoporosis.

Our understanding of how the mind works and how our emotions affect our body's function has been demonstrated without question, and even though we are still searching for the answer to the ultimate question of our existence we have enough technologies available for emotional and spiritual growth. The more we develop emotionally and spiritually the more chances we have to heal, reduce our suffering and live happier, productive and profound lives.

We hope this book will provide information that will give you the knowledge and insight; and the basis to strengthen your motivation to heal and develop hope about the future. Only you are able to strengthen your will through practice as you develop the positive habits that will lead you to a more fulfilling life, as free of disease as is possible.

Bernardo Merizalde, M.D.

Foreword

I never paid much attention to all the articles and news reports on bone health. Let me re-phrase that. I paid attention; I just had no personal stake in it. Of course, I wanted to be informed for the seminars I taught, so that I could provide people with the most up-to-date information. But I lived a healthy vegan lifestyle, exercising regularly and eating very well. My husband, a distance runner was just as healthy, so I paid attention only from a philosophical standpoint.

That all changed in 1998, when Robert, at age 48, was diagnosed with severe osteoporosis. To say that we were shocked would be the understatement of the century, particularly with his secondary diagnosis . . . severe malnutrition. His symptoms were acute and painful, with stress fracture after stress fracture plaguing his existence. After careful reflection and tons of research, we came to the conclusion that we could manage his condition with diet and supplementation, that pharmaceuticals were not the answer for us.

Now for those of you who know my history and my work, this will not surprise you. I had cured my own case of cancer (leukemia, to be exact) back in 1983 with an austere macrobiotic diet, which ironically, turned out to be the long-term problem for us. Let me explain. When I was curing my cancer, my husband and I embraced a strict macrobiotic style of cooking and eating, designed to regain my health, which obviously worked, since I am still here, living a healthy, fulfilling life. We went wrong, though, continuing this monastic 'healing diet' approach to eating for many years after my recovery. Our diet was very low in both fat and protein, and while rich in whole grains, seasonal vegetables and fruit, nuts and seeds, it was not appropriate for our level of activity, resulting in feeling and being malnourished.

We consulted with our family doctor, Bernardo Merizalde, M.D. and came up with a plan for Robert that included various supplements and homeopathic remedies, as well as a revamping of our diet. Using the wisdom I gained from many years of macrobiotic practice and Chinese medicine, as well as my masters degree in food nutrition, we altered our eating patterns, designing a plan for us

15

that increased the intake of good quality fats (we practically drink olive oil now) and protein, including fish (for Robert, not me . . . I still choose to be vegan). The result? Well, you will read his amazing story in this book, but let me just say that he has fully recovered. No pharmaceuticals of any kind were required. It took four years, but he is back to distance running, free of pain and has shown unprecedented bone re-growth.

I have learned a lot from this experience, improving both my husband's and my health and once again I am moved by the power of food choices in our health and well-being. For me, facing a crisis is an opportunity to grow and learn. After the initial shock, I am motivated to action, which usually begins with research, so I can understand what is going on. It is with information that we can make educated choices and will not act from ignorance and fear. It is with information that we can regain our power and become a proactive partner in regaining and maintaining our health.

My husband is an amazing man, as you will see in this book. He is a man of passion, dedication, loyalty, integrity and honesty. He is the man who has made all of my dreams come true. He is the man who, after more than twenty-two years of life together, still has me catching the breath he takes away. He is the man who, at the end of the day, when I slip between the sheets and snuggle to his side, completes me.

Read what he has to say in these pages . . . it's a story of hope, recovery, determination and the power of love.

Christina Pirello

Introduction

Why I Wrote this Book

If you are reading this book, you no doubt are either suffering with osteoporosis, suspect you have osteoporosis, are a care giver for somebody with osteoporosis, or want to do everything you possibly can to prevent being diagnosed with osteoporosis. You may have also looked at other books on the subject, done research on-line, and most likely talked with a medical professional.

What makes this book different? Unlike other books on the subject, *B.O.N.E.S.* delves into the effects our dietary choices have on the cause, prevention and cure of osteoporosis. It also provides a primer, in laymen's terms, for understanding your bones and osteoporosis, as well as your risk factors for developing this silent disease. It takes into consideration that no two people are alike. Two people, with identical diagnoses may, in fact, have totally different symptoms. And these same two people will handle their diagnosis differently from both an emotional and treatment standpoint. It also looks into the psychological impact of dealing with chronic disease, as well as exploring both alternative and conventional therapies to regaining bone density. In addition, it provides guidelines to assist you in making an appropriate treatment decision.

Let's face it . . . we're all getting older, and we're doing it faster than at any other period in the history of human civilization. And not only are we getting older, but we're staying alive longer. Unfortunately we're doing it at a very high cost, because contrary to popular belief, we're not staying alive longer in a healthy way. The trends in aging and the condition of our health as we age and the implications of those trends are staggering.

In February 2002, the United Nations released data and startling statistics on global population aging. Here are just a few statistics:

Projected growth in numbers of persons age 60 plus:

2002:   1 in 10 persons
2050:   1 in 5 persons

Projected growth in the percentage of age 65 plus bracket, over the age of 85:

2002:   12%
2050:   21%

Projected growth in number of centenarians (people age 100 and over):

2002:   210,000 worldwide
2050:   312 million worldwide (a fifteen-fold increase)

Average global life expectancy at birth has climbed nearly 20 years since 1950, to stand at 66 years old. Improvements in science, healthcare, preventative health, nutrition and sanitation have all translated into falling mortality rates. It is predicted that global mortality will drop faster in the next 20 years than previously in the last decade.

Think about that for a moment. That means that more older people will be alive than at any time before. The UN also predicts that by 2050, the number of people age 60 and over will outnumber that of children, to stand at 2 billion worldwide.

The U.S. population currently stands at 300 million. Approximately 12%—35 million—are age 65 and over. This age bracket will swell enormously with the aging of the Baby Boomer population (those born between 1946 and 1964), 76 million strong. Since 1990, the number of 45 to 54 year olds (representing the first half of the Baby Boomer generation), has jumped a remarkable 49%.

In 2011, the first of the Baby Boomer generation begins to turn 65 years old. As a result, by 2030, 1 in 5 Americans will be at least that old. The size of the older population is projected to double over the next 30 years, growing to 70 million by 2030. When we rang in the new millennium, we also shattered previous records for U.S. life expectancy. In May 2002, the U.S. Center for Disease Control, (CDC), reported that as of 2000, U.S. life expectancy hit an all-time high with an average of 76.9 years. Babies born in 2002 are expected to live well into their mid to late eighties.

What have all these statistics to do with your bones? While the UN study enlightened us on aging statistics, it did little to inform us on how poor dietary habits are currently affecting us as we age.

The study did show us that collectively, chronic diseases account for 70% of all deaths in the U.S. And medical costs for people with chronic diseases account for more than 60% of the nation's medical care costs. In 2000 alone, treatment of osteoporosis cost us more than $14 billion . . . billion, with a 'B.'

As we look at this staggering number, the first question we should be asking ourselves is, how much of chronic diseases like osteoporosis are preventable? Equally important, how much of it is self-inflicted as a result of poor dietary practices?

This is our wake-up call. At this rate we will no doubt be living longer and longer, but in poorer and poorer health. And who is going to foot the bill? Medical costs and health insurance are already beyond the reach of many, and these costs are not going down; they're only going up. The implications for our economy, and our very way of life are staggering.

Look around; we're fat, out of shape, and the willing victims of marketing. We live in a land of excess. Walking into a supermarket today is like walking into 'Disneyland;' there isn't anything we can't have . . . or get. At the same time, we no longer know how to nourish ourselves properly. Consider this . . . generally speaking the baby boomer generation is the last generation that knows how to create a complete balanced meal from scratch, whether they choose to or not. The generation that follows knows what a balanced meal should look like, and can assemble one from prepared purchased foods. The generation that follows thinks a healthy, balanced meal is a 'Happy Meal' that comes with bottled water and a pedometer.

A major step toward putting an end to this madness is through education. Exercise needs to become a part of our daily routine, as does getting back into the kitchen and learning to cook and nourish ourselves once again. Let's face it, we're all familiar with that little voice in our heads that says, "there's a better choice," as we reach for that soda or candy bar. Don't you find it interesting that 'junk food' is part of our vocabulary? Is it really that difficult to make the connection between the decline in the condition of our overall health as a culture over the past four decades and the food we choose to eat? Do we really need to spend billions of dollars on research to determine why so many of our children are obese and beginning to suffer from heart disease, adult onset diabetes, even arthritis in their teenage years? Our children are in this condition from lack of physical activity and too much soda and junk food.

And osteoporosis? Not far-fetched for our children, either. Only 14% of girls and 36% of boys age 12 to 19 in the U.S. are getting the recommended amounts of calcium, according to the USDA. Close to 90% of adult bone is established by the end of the teen years. So if kids are off to a bad start in getting enough calcium, says the National Institute of Child Health and Human Development, they are at serious risk of developing osteoporosis as well as other bone diseases down the road. These statistics were all motivating factors in writing this book.

The biggest difference between this and any other book on the subject is that this is my story. In 1998, at the age of 48, I was diagnosed with severe osteoporosis. I was told I had the bones of an 86-year-old man; and I felt like I had the bones of an 86-year-old man. So what's so unusual about that you may ask? First, I'm a man and men don't get osteoporosis; women do, or so we are led to believe. Secondly, I've been a health advocate all of my life. I'd done everything right, or so I thought, from diet to exercise . . . all designed to maintain an optimal level of health. Before you turn to the last page, allow me to tell you how the story ends. I've been successful in regaining substantial bone density and reversing severe osteoporosis and I did it with a natural alternative approach that I detail in this book. But when I stop and think about why I felt compelled to write all this down, there are obvious and not so obvious reasons.

The most obvious reason is that osteoporosis is a major public health threat for more than 44 million Americans aged 50 and older. More than 10 million people in the United States already have osteoporosis, and that number is rapidly growing with the graying of America. Another 34 million people have low bone mass, placing them at increased risk of osteoporosis fractures in the future, and with the rapidly aging population, these numbers will continue to increase at a staggering rate.

The not so obvious reasons for writing this book? The misconception that osteoporosis is a disease that affects only women, when in fact, one third of all hip fractures, and hip replacements caused by osteoporosis occur in men. Add to that the fact that early signs of osteoporosis are showing up in more and more young adults everyday. There is no doubt osteoporosis will become a major concern for our youth.

While our bones (as well as many of our other parts), are deteriorating at a rapid rate, we are obsessed with staying and looking young, at any cost. We are bombarded with and seduced by messages promoting products that promise to reverse aging. Staying young has become a multi-billion dollar business. Both pharmaceutical manufacturers and natural food companies are out to convince us that they have the key to "the fountain of youth." The true challenge that we all face is not staying young forever, (we're all going to get old), but rather living a long, productive, fulfilling, healthy life.

Our greatest gift is the gift of life. With it comes great responsibility, first to ourselves; we must love ourselves and take care of ourselves. In this life we have but one body; yet for the most part we give it very little thought. In many instances, we take better care of our cars and other possessions than we do of our bodies. Secondly, we have a responsibility to one and other. We must love one another; we must care for and look after one another, and we must do so as if our lives depended on it—because they do.

I wrote this book because I care.

Robert Pirello

Part One

All About Osteoporosis

Chapter 1

An Unlikely Victim

MY STORY OF "O"STEOPOROSIS

Running and Being

Sunday, November 2, 1997, New York, New York, the greatest city in the world. There I was at eight o'clock in the morning, on Staten Island with thirty-thousand like-minded people from all over the world, filled with the excitement and anticipation of running the 20th annual New York City Marathon. It's hard to describe the feeling and emotion of the moment. The energy on the island is electrifying. Imagine thousands of people with a single goal, running 26.2 miles, from the base of the Verrazano Bridge in Staten Island to Tavern on the Green in Central Park, passing through all five boroughs of New York City in the process.

This would be my twelfth New York City marathon and each time it amazes me. It is quite the spectacle; people from every walk of life, from actors and actresses to TV personalities and corporate executives, to elite athletes and weekend warriors, all will run together toward one goal, one common dream . . . crossing that finish line 26.2 miles away.

Over the years of running the race, I'd run through every kind of weather imaginable, from frigid cold to unseasonably hot. But most years, early November in The Big Apple is pretty pleasant, with temperatures in the 50's, perfect marathon weather. This particular marathon Sunday was rather dreary and dismal, not cold, but the air thick with humidity, dark and gray with the threat of heavy rain looming in the air. While the front runners would most likely beat the rain, us middle-of-the-packers were no doubt going to get plenty wet. "If only the race could start now," I thought at eight o'clock, "perhaps I could beat the rain." But the starting cannon would not sound for another three hours.

Marathon day is completely different than any of your training runs. It's easy to get caught up in the crowd and the excitement of the moment and go out too fast; you can easily lose it and hit the wall between twenty-two and twenty-three miles, in which case, the last miles can seem like an eternity. It's often said that the marathon begins at mile twenty-two. I've been known to joke that mile twenty-three is when most men experience childbirth. I had no idea how right I would be this year . . . and how different this marathon would be for me . . . and how my life was about to change.

At about 10:00AM, the herding process began as runners started the mass exodus from the Staten Island grounds to the base of the Verrazano Bridge, finding their appropriate starting stall based on their anticipated finishing time. In nervous anticipation of the starting cannon, attempting to listen to a litany of speeches under the chatter of the crowd and the whir of countless helicopters in the sky above, you can hear a pin drop as the national anthem is sung, followed by thundering applause, the blast of the starting cannon and the sound of 30,000 feet as they began their 26.2 mile journey to Tavern on the Green in Central Park.

The first eighteen or so miles of the marathon are usually pretty uneventful for a well-trained marathoner, who will prepare over a period of four to six months, building strength and stamina day by day, week by week, month by month. My own marathon strategy has always been to run the first 10K (6.2 miles), and the last 10K at the same pace, so all I had to do was run approximately fourteen miles in the middle. And anyone can run fourteen miles, right?

I considered myself the picture of health, until the summer of 1997, well into my training for my twelfth New York City Marathon. Having run over twenty marathons, I knew my body pretty well and I sensed something was wrong; something was very wrong. But I couldn't put my finger on what it was that plagued me, but I can recall the feeling like it was yesterday.

Having been a runner for most of my adult life, averaging between forty and fifty miles a week, clocking as many as one hundred miles a week in my early marathon days, I had never felt like this. I was haunted by a very deep inner weakness I had never experienced before, a weakness that I felt with each and every step, like it went to my very core. I was having a difficult time breathing during hard training runs and my ribs would scream with pain on the downhill treks. Running, something that came very natural to me, had become a tremendous effort. Most of the time, I felt extremely fragile and fatigued.

I struggled through the summer of 1997 and with it, my worst marathon training season ever; but November 2nd arrived, and there I was . . . at the starting line of the New York City Marathon. I stood there listening to the national anthem and for the first time in all my years of running, I questioned whether or not I had the strength and stamina to complete the 26.2 mile course, a course I could run with my eyes closed . . . a course I had run over and over in my head, countless number of times with great anticipation.

There was no quitting now. The singer sang, ". . . . and the land of the brave." The cannon fired, and we took off, 30,000 strong. The humidity was relentless, but the first miles passed quickly. I hit the half way point, feeling pretty weak and tired. Could it have been the humidity or was it more of the same fatigue and weakness I had been experiencing for the past several months?

At the twenty mile mark there was a huge flash of lightning followed by a crash of thunder. As I ran through the Bronx, the sky opened up with torrential wind-swept rain that would continue through the rest of the day and evening. The rain came down in sheets so hard that you could barely see your hand in front of your face. The wind was blowing me sideways throughout most of the last six miles. The streets were suddenly flooded. In some places the water was ankle deep. The finish line, usually a gala party, was uneventful, and my worst marathon finishing time ever. In the pouring rain, wind and now cold temperatures, I slowly walked back to my hotel. A hot shower, a good dinner, and a good night's sleep were what I needed now. I'd be fine, or so I thought.

My Inspiration

I began running March 1, 1976. I was almost twenty-seven years old. My running career had its beginnings in a very strange and almost mystical way. I was driving home from work on February 28 and stopped at a convenience store to buy a bag of potato chips and a carton of cigarettes, (I smoked three, sometimes four packs a day and weighed fifty pounds more than I should have). As I approached my street and prepared to make a left turn, I saw him coming toward me. He was running, shirtless, wearing a pair of blue running shorts, his long blond hair blowing in the breeze. What's so unusual about that? Well, it was the end of February, and while a common sight today, this was 1976 and I lived in Harrisburg, Pennsylvania. I had never seen anything like him before. It seemed to me that he had fallen from the sky . . . or perhaps he was from California, I thought at the time. Those were my actual thoughts at that moment. Seeing him stirred something very deep within me. It was a very surreal moment.

I went home, put the carton of cigarettes in my nightstand drawer (not realizing that I would quit smoking the very next day). I couldn't get the image of this running man out of my mind. The next morning I woke up early, put on a pair of old pants, a sweatshirt, my winter coat and tennis shoes and ran out my front door. I think I ran a single block before doubling over, feeling like I was coughing up a lung. But in an odd way, something felt right about it. So it began . . . each and every day I would get up early to run and walk. I would also park my car a mile from my office and walk the rest of the way to work.

At lunch, I would walk some more. It took me a month to work up to running a mile nonstop, then two miles, followed by three. Before I know it, I was running at least six miles a day, and walking another three or four.

Six months later, I was a new person. My life had changed forever. I had lost fifty pounds, had an amazing positive attitude about . . . everything. Even my diet did a complete three-sixty. I realized that on the road of life, good health is a lifelong pursuit, and my life could not have been better. I realized too, that running was a form of play that brought out the kid in me, and it made every day a new adventure. I had discovered my fountain of youth. When people would ask me what I 'did' for a living, my response was always, "I'm a runner."

For the next twenty-one years I considered myself to be pretty invincible. There was nothing I wouldn't take on . . . and nothing I couldn't conquer. When it came to my running, my skill and stamina continued to improve. I was competing in races of all distances, and I ran them fast and furious, clocking enviable times for each distance, including a full 26.2-mile marathon in two hours and forty-three minutes. I was a runner . . . that is, until 1997, when it all began to change.

It All Started in Barbados . . .

After the New York City Marathon of 1997, I made the conscious decision to take some time off from running and see if I could figure out what was going on with my health. I wanted to regain my strength, and get back to being my old self. Little did I know what was in store for me. Over the next couple of months, still feeling week and fragile, I cut back on my running, but I was looking forward to our annual winter getaway to Barbados.

My wife Christina and I have a travel company that we founded in 1989. We organize and host healthy vacations, taking intimate groups of guests on wonderful holidays to Europe and the Caribbean, providing healthy meals, as well as touring, hiking and sailing We would be in Barbados for two weeks in February 1998 with guests joining us for one of the two weeks . . . and a holiday for us during the second.

Arriving in Barbados in advance of the group, I did a little running on the island, but remained haunted by this weak, fragile feeling that just wouldn't lift. I had planned a full-day hike through the rainforest for the group, with me as their fearless leader. It would prove to be quite an adventure, as well as the day that would begin a new chapter in my life.

The hike itself was quite fun, although a bit treacherous, even by my standards. We had to lower ourselves by vines down the side of steep inclines in some areas, pull ourselves up in other areas. In the last hour of the hike, we were walking on trails that were a little rocky, but pretty flat, so I decided to run ahead of the group a short distance. About a half mile ahead of the group, I stepped on a rock and twisted my foot. Throbbing pain immediately engulfed my entire foot and ankle, followed by swelling and a lovely shade of black and blue. When the group finally caught up to me, I was totally immobile. I could not walk or even stand on my foot without excruciating pain. The guides had to carry me a short distance to where a vehicle could navigate into the jungle and pick me up. I was in pain and now humiliated.

Turns out, I had broken my left foot, the fifth metatarsal, to be exact. I struggled through that night in pain so excruciating it brought tears to my eyes. I spent the better part of the next day (while Christina tended to the responsibility of the trip and the guests) at a hospital in Barbados having x-rays and an old-fashioned plaster cast put on my foot . . . a cast that weighed almost as much as I did.

Pain aside, I thought nothing of it. I figured I would get back home to Philadelphia, make an appointment with an orthopedic doctor; the cast would be off in four weeks. I'd go through a little physical therapy and be back running in no time. I had no idea that I would not run for nearly two and a half years and that once I did start running, I would be diagnosed with compression fractures in all five lumbar vertebrae and suffer a series of stress fractures in just about every joint in my body. I now understand the cliché that says, 'it's better we don't know what lies ahead.'

The balance of the trip was quite a struggle, attempting to get around on crutches. And it would be twelve days before I would be back home and able to properly tend to my broken foot. The pain was relentless. You know how the time seems to fly by when you're on vacation? Well, these proved to be twelve of the longest days of my life.

The Pain of Healing

Back home in Philadelphia, I called the Foot and Ankle Institute and set up an appointment to have the damage surveyed by an orthopedic physician. New x-rays of my foot detected not one, but three breaks. My anticipated four weeks in a cast, according to my doctors, would be six weeks, beginning with two weeks in a temporary 'Jones' cast, which allowed for icing to bring down massive swelling from the plaster cast put on my foot in Barbados. Then, I would wear a more permanent cast for another four weeks.

Having already been in a cast for nearly two weeks, with this diagnosis, that would mean I would be in a cast for a total of eight weeks. But I figured I could live with that; it would force me not to run and perhaps the rest would do me good.

We runners, however, are a stubborn bunch. Once the permanent cast went on, I took it easy for a couple of days, but not being able to run got the best of me. I decided to try running on crutches. I mean, why not? I went out every day, running as fast as I could, crutches and all. I was actually feeling pretty good. I figured running with crutches would make me stronger, and make it easier to start up my running regimen once the permanent cast came off.

Two weeks after putting on the permanent cast, I was surprised when they cut it off to take new x-rays. The new x-rays showed no improvement. "What?" I thought, "six weeks have gone by and my foot is no better?" A new cast was put on and I left with an appointment for two weeks later. Over the next two weeks, I continued running every day, working up to five miles. At the doctor's office two weeks later, new x-rays again showed no improvement.

At this point, the baffled doctor asked me what I was doing. She could not understand why I was not healing. After all, it had now been eight weeks. Even I thought I'd be totally healed, out of the cast, and running on two legs again. Instead, the break was not mending at all. So I told her everything I did during my day. Then I got to the part about running every day. Let's just say that it didn't go over very well. She explained to me that I had to sit with my foot elevated just about all the time if I wanted it to heal. Running was in fact causing the foot to bounce around and thus not heal. Okay, that made sense. Now I was faced with being in a cast for yet another four weeks, bringing my total cast time to three months. Talk about depressed!

For the next two weeks, I behaved myself and went to the doctor quite hopeful. To my dismay, the x-rays showed that the break was a little better, but not promising enough to think that the cast would come off permanently in anther two weeks. It continued like this for five months, yes, five months; I wore a cast from mid-February to mid-July before my foot was healed sufficiently to remove the cast for good.

Once the cast was off, my left calf, much to my dismay, was half the size of my right, *and my foot still hurt!* It seemed as if I had to learn to walk all over again. And running? I couldn't even think about running. Okay, to be honest, all I did was think about running; I dreamed about running. I didn't know if I'd ever run again. I was really depressed. I was used to endorphin rushes and dopamine highs. Now all I did is sit around and dream about running.

My Osteoporosis Diagnosis

With my leg free from its cast, I began walking, albeit gingerly. I walked as much as possible, and I did a little strength training in an attempt to restore my atrophied left calf muscle. In September, two months after the cast was removed, I made my first attempt at running. I ran like a little old man, all hunched over, favoring my weak leg, half running, half limping. I was a sorry sight. Within a very short time, about two weeks after beginning running, I began to realize severe pain in my lower back that wrapped around my lower rib cage. Pain that kept me awake at night. Pain that woke me up in a cold sweat. Pain that I felt when I stepped off of a curb. Pain so intense that I had to pull myself up steps one at a time, while holding on to the banister. Pain that brought tears to my eyes. Pain like I had never experienced. Pain that caused me to call the pain clinic at Jefferson Hospital. I had to get to the bottom of this for once and for all. Why did I break my foot? Why did it take five months to heal? Why was I tired and fatigued all the time? Why was I in agonizing pain all the time? What was going on? It was time to find out!

The appointment at Jefferson was uneventful with one major exception. After examining me, the doctor suggested I have an x-ray of my spine, which we did right then and there. Back in the examining room, observing my x-ray, he said, "I think I see some osteoporosis."

I immediately wrote off this suggestion; in fact I didn't even give it a second thought, because I knew he was wrong. However, I agreed to a DEXA scan the following week in order to rule out this absurd notion that I could possibly have osteoporosis.

I will never forget the day. It was October 12, 1998, just 7:00am, when the phone rang. I was shaving, getting ready to head off to work: Christina was still fast asleep. Startled by the early call, I answered.

"Good morning, Mr. Pirello?," I immediately recognized the voice of the doctor from Jefferson Hospital. What he was about to tell me would change the course of my life . . . for the rest of my life. It would make me question choices that I thought were healthy diet and lifestyle choices I had made over the past thirty-years of my life.

"Mr. Pirello, the results of your DEXA scan are in," he said, rather matter-of-factly; and bluntly to the point, "you have severe osteoporosis. You have the bones of an eighty-six year old man." Some news for 7:00 in the morning!

As he was speaking, my mind reeled with all kinds of thoughts and questions: 'men don't get osteoporosis; it's a woman's disease; what about my running . . . will I ever be able to run again; this is a misdiagnosis; I'll get a second opinion. Are my bones going to start breaking randomly; will my wife be pushing me around in a wheel chair before I turn fifty; I eat a healthy diet that claims to prevent osteoporosis; what's up with that?' and on and on?

"Call my office after 9:00am," the doctor continued, "to set up an appointment. I'd also like you to see a rheumatologist. I'll recommend a couple for you to choose from. I also want to refer you to a sports medicine orthopedic surgeon." I assumed he wanted me to see a sports medicine doctor since I had been a dedicated, (well, to be completely honest, fanatical), athlete for most of my life. I hung up the phone in complete and utter shock.

Boy, Was I Depressed . . . and Scared

"You have severe osteoporosis." At that moment, I understood what it felt like to be run down by a speeding truck or to fall down an elevator shaft from the two-hundredth floor of a skyscraper. While not a death sentence, all I could visualize was my skeleton, my very foundation, the strongest part of my physical being degenerating, crumbling, and becoming extremely fragile at a very young age. And all I could imagine was living a life of severe, chronic pain, with the constant fear of fracturing every bone in my body. After all, for the past several months, my pain, on a scale of one to ten, was somewhere in the neighborhood of, oh . . . ten thousand.

I got in and out of a car with great difficulty; had to pre-plan how I would get up from a seated position prior to sitting down on a sofa or chair, and I could forget about rolling over in bed in the middle of the night, or getting out of bed first thing in the morning! Many a night I would awaken sobbing from the intensity of the pain.

I experienced severe back and hip pain simply stepping off of a curb. I would soon discover, as a result of an MRI, that all of my pain was caused by compression fractures of all five lumbar vertebrae and spontaneous recurring stress fractures of both hips, my left knee, right foot, and several ribs. To say I was depressed would be an understatement, but at least now I knew the cause of my pain, and could now put my energy toward discovering its cause and beginning the healing process.

An Unlikely Candidate

Before going any further, allow me to put a few things into perspective. First and foremost, I thought myself to be the picture of health. In addition to being a marathon runner, I had been practicing and living a macrobiotic lifestyle for nearly thirty years, eating practically no meat or animal products, with the exception of an occasional piece of fish. My diet was largely based on whole grains, beans, soyfoods, whole wheat pasta, and lots and lots of vegetables, (including sea vegetables for their high mineral content). And now, at the age of forty-eight, I was being told that I had the bones of an eighty-six year old man. This could not really be happening, but it really was!

One of my first thoughts was that it could be genetic, but based on my family history, I was a most unlikely candidate for osteoporosis. My mother was one of fifteen children, my father one of five. My grandparents on both sides were hearty Sicilian immigrants. My grandmother on my mother's side gave birth to two sets of twins, her first born and her last born (at the age of 49). I have a huge extended family. In fact one of our little jokes is that we rent the state of Rhode Island for family gatherings. We are also a very closely knit family, so it was not difficult for me to research my family history for osteoporosis. What I found shocked me. I could not find a single diagnosis of osteoporosis anywhere in my immediate or extended family. Not one, so why me?

Growing up, while a little weird, I was a really healthy active kid. Weird, because, being of Italian heritage, I didn't really like traditional Italian food and was always nosing around in 'health food stores.' I was always out playing and bike riding. I played tennis in high school, almost fanatically. And I began running in my late twenties. For the life of me, I could not come up with a single clue as to how I could be a candidate for osteoporosis.

The Christina Factor

I wasn't quite sure what to tell Christina that morning in October, but I had to tell her something. As I stood there still holding the phone in my hand, she sat up in bed and asked, "Who was on the phone?" I gave her the news as it was relayed to me, and somehow, in the disbelief and confusion of it all, continued getting ready for the day.

Allow me a minute to tell you a bit about Christina. I met my wife in June of 1983. At the time, she had just been diagnosed with AML, an acute form of leukemia, and given a prognosis of six to nine months to live. Not sure what she would do, at the ripe young age of 27, a mutual friend, (knowing my interest and experience in macrobiotics), introduced us. We, of course, hit it off, and Christina decided to give macrobiotics a go, while her doctors monitored her blood on a regular basis. Much to everyone's surprise . . . and delight . . . months ticked by and Christina was still hanging around. During this process, we fell in love. Fourteen months after practicing and eating macrobiotically, Christina was declared leukemia-free. We celebrated her health and future and eventually we were married . . . and today, over twenty years later, we are in the process of living happily ever after . . .

Christina and I talked over breakfast that morning. She was as shocked as I was by my diagnosis. Here she was, a cancer survivor, a noted healthy cooking show host on PBS, and author of healthy lifestyle cookbooks. Like me, she didn't know what to think, but one thing was certain, we were determined to get more information, find the cause and decide on a course of action. Her expertise, with regard to nutrition and the power of food in healing would be put to use once again.

The Shocking Truth

Not one to run to a doctor every time I experience an ache or pain, at that moment I had to rely on medical professionals in an effort to determine the cause of my osteoporosis and to come up with an appropriate treatment. I went for my follow up visit to the doctor. This time I left with four prescriptions, one for an MRI of my spine, another for a complete blood work-up, another for a twenty-four hour urinalysis, and one more for a referral follow-up visit with a sports medicine physician.

Much to my surprise, the results of my blood work and urinalysis were normal. The results of my MRI, on the other hand were beyond mind-boggling, and would send me into a state of utter confusion and depression like I had never known. I remember the sports medicine orthopedic surgeon backing away from the MRI of my spine lit up on the wall, mumbling to himself, "Oh my God, oh my God, I have never seen anything like this before."

He proceeded to tell me that I had compression fractures of all five lumbar, and that my spine looked like something out of a deprived Third World country. And then he dropped a major bomb. The cause of my osteoporosis.

He told me that I was suffering from a severe case of malnutrition. Talk about shocking truth. This doctor gave me three more prescriptions. The first was to see a nutritionist, the second was for Fosamax (a pharmaceutical commonly used to treat osteoporosis), and third was for fifteen weeks of physical therapy. This was getting scarier by the minute. Malnutrition? I'm 'Mr. Health Food'. I'm an athlete who eats enormous amounts of food. How could I be malnourished?

Christina, like me, didn't know what to think or do, but as she had done when she was diagnosed with cancer all those years ago, would not stand idly by. She knew that our answers would come from research, but in the meantime we had to take some action. At that moment, Christina made a suggestion that would be yet another turning point in my story. Before seeing a nutritionist, taking Fosamax or going into physical therapy, she suggested I call Bernardo Merizalde, a homeopathic M.D. she had worked with over the years when she experienced any problems that required medical attention; and since she had just recently suffered a major health setback and worked with Dr. Merizalde once again, he was fresh in her mind and at the top of her list for help.

The Year From Hell

We all have them from time to time . . . periods in our lives when nothing seems to go right, and if one more thing goes wrong, you don't know what you will do. We call it a string of bad luck. Well, 1998 was our year from hell. The straw that broke the camel's back kept coming and coming . . . there was no one 'straw.' We had bales of straws that year. I broke my foot in February. Two months later in April, Christina suffered a brain aneurysm that would land her in the neuro-trauma unit at University of Pennsylvania Hospital, (which we would later learn was diet-related as well), and I was diagnosed with severe osteoporosis caused by malnutrition.

We prayed for New Year's Day. 1999 couldn't come fast enough. We were in need of a change in luck. Through all of this we had to figure out a way to get on with our lives. We had a business to run. Christina was in the middle of writing her third book, teaching cooking classes, producing a new series of "Christina Cooks" for PBS; we had trips scheduled and a magazine to publish. In addition, I had a full time job working for an advertising agency. We had to work. So we struggled through it, me with my crutches and brittle bones and Christina with a constant headache and a pool of blood at the base of her brain. But we had each other and that gave us strength.

Meeting Dr. Merizalde

While Christina had seen Dr. Merizalde professionally on many occasions, I had not. My first encounter with the good doctor was a lengthy telephone conversation, which I found quite amazing since I had never had a doctor spend so much time with me on the telephone prior to seeing me. Dr. Merizalde had many professional questions and requested I get him copies of all my recent medical records prior to our first appointment.

If I was amazed by that first encounter, my first appointment blew me away. Anybody who has been to a doctor knows the drill. You call and make an appointment; usually get one a month from the time you call. You don't talk to the doctor until the day of your appointment. On the day of your visit, you arrive early in order to fill out pages of documents, and then you wait, (usually well past your appointment time), to see the doctor. Once in the examining room you wait some more, and usually you'll see an intern or physicians assistant prior to seeing the doctor who may spend ten or fifteen minutes with you . . . on a good day.

Arriving at Dr. Merizalde's office for my first appointment, I wasn't quite sure what to expect, but the experience turned out to be much different than any other doctor's appointment I had ever had. Dr. Merizalde spent nearly two hours with me. By the end of the visit, he had made numerous observations and suggestions based on my medical history, family history, current medical diagnosis and condition, medical records, lifestyle, and so very much more. His primary recommendations included a regimen that included homeopathic remedies, supplementation, physical therapy, and a modified exercise program. For the moment he suggested holding off on taking Fosamax.

Christina's Research Pays Off

Christina's research also began to pay off . . . big time . . . we had a clear answer to the most baffling question of all, "How could I be malnourished?" After spending numerous hours online researching osteoporosis, the incidence of osteoporosis in men, women and athletes, Christina found a connection between my monastic macrobiotic diet of nearly thirty years, and my addiction to running for over twenty years.

It seems that osteoporosis is prevalent in many athletes who run and/or cycle. The incidence increases when you factor in certain dietary patterns, especially those that restrict dietary fat and protein, which a strict macrobiotic diet does. Fat is required for energy production and to supply essential fatty acids and fat-soluble vitamins (A, D, E, K). Protein is required to build muscle tissue. The research was decisive . . . restricting and/or avoiding all foods that contain fat and protein reduces the variety of foods eaten and can lead to nutritional deficiencies. The message was coming through loud and clear; I had to make major dietary changes.

Now, before you assume that this book is not for you because you are not an athlete and you don't eat a macrobiotic diet, guess again. For over twenty-five years, in an unsuccessful effort to reduce the waistline of America, low-fat diets were advised as part of healthy, balanced eating. While the food message today is NO or LOW CARB, for several decades the diet craze was NO or LOW FAT! Everything in the supermarket was labeled "FAT FREE". The resulting effect has been devastating; we're only still fat, but obesity has become a major epidemic; and osteoporosis is on the rise. And this trend is still in vogue today.

The information on fat then was clearly bad information, just as the information on carbohydrates today is bad information. Instead of attacking all fat, we should have focused on reducing saturated fat. Today instead of attacking all carbs, we should be attacking simple, refined carbohydrates. As a result, many people, (and clearly many women, mostly affected by osteoporosis), did not and continue to not consume enough healthy dietary fat and essential fatty acids in order to assimilate fat-soluble nutrients. Add to this the fact that most people do not consume the required amounts of many essential nutrients. And we don't exercise. Only 19% of Americans get regular weight-bearing exercise. It's no wonder osteoporosis is rampant today.

The Next Several Years

After much contemplation and self-reflection, what became clear to me was that I made certain choices in my life that resulted in my being diagnosed with osteoporosis. The next several years were clearly not going to be easy. My condition was serious. It would take time, but I was convinced that I could restore my health while regaining bone density.

What gave me the most hope and conviction was something my osteoporosis doctor at Jefferson Hospital in Philadelphia said to me. While attempting to convince me to take Fosamax, he explained to me that bone was living tissue and that you get a whole new skeleton every three to four years. "Wow," I remember thinking, "if that's the case, why not put all of my energy for the next three years towards building a 'healthy' new skeleton." A bit simplistic, but I figured I had nothing to lose; the next three years would go by anyway.

I was right. It was not easy. I spoke with Dr. Merizalde via phone on occasion, saw him for several follow up visits, and took the indicated supplements and homeopathic remedies. I also saw my osteoporosis doctor at Jefferson Hospital for annual DEXA scans, (something I continue to do), and blood and urinalysis testing. I did the fifteen weeks of physical therapy, and also worked with a sports medicine doctor at Temple University Hospital, as needed, in order to get back to running. And while I saw progress, (I did, in fact, gain some bone density as opposed to losing it), I was still plagued by numerous setbacks in the form of recurring spontaneous stress fractures in my hips, feet and knees. I would run for eight to twelve weeks and then I'd be down for eight to twelve weeks with a stress fracture. It seemed as though one would pop up every few months. As a result, I had more MRI's and bone scans than one could imagine, but I was persistent and determined. I would run another marathon.

As a result of dietary changes, (mostly adding good quality fat and protein to my regular daily diet), over the next eight to twelve months, I gained a much needed twenty-five pounds, and overall, I looked and felt better. But I still felt like there was something missing . . . something that could help me to strengthen my bones and joints in order to stop the stress fractures. I continued to feel somewhat fragile when I ran, never knowing when the next stress fracture would occur and where. I continued to search the Internet for an answer. An answer I would eventually find.

My Turning Point

Three years had passed since my original diagnosis in October of 1998. It was November 2001. I was sitting at my computer searching the web, when I came upon a clinical study on the effects of red yeast rice (a product readily available in most natural foods stores) on osteoporosis. The study claimed that certain strains of red yeast rice could build bone density in osteoporotic bone, and could do so five-fold, in as little as twelve to sixteen weeks.

Okay, I was game. I sent away for a product that had been certified bone active an independent laboratory in Texas and began taking the product, along with a daily regimen of supplements, immediately. After fourteen weeks I was scheduled for my annual DEXA scan. The results floored both Dr. Merizalde and me. He called, as well as faxed me a copy of the report from Jefferson Hospital. He was so excited he was nearly jumping through the phone line. As in previous years, DEXA scans of my lumbar spine and left hip were obtained. In previous years, I had shown marked improvement, but the process of healing was slow. This time, the bone density interval in my lumbar spine showed an increase of 9.4%. In my hip, the interval increase was 6.6%. The report stated that this was "a significant, unprecedented increase."

For me, the most striking change was that I no longer felt the least bit fragile or hesitant. I began to feel stronger and sturdier; and more significantly, since November 2001 to the present, I have not suffered a single stress fracture recurrence.

November 3, 2002

If 1998 was the year from hell, 2002 was a new beginning and to celebrate, I decided I would train for the New York City Marathon in November. While my body once again felt strong, my mind was still a bit hesitant. After all, I hadn't run a marathon in five years. I carefully planned my training schedule. I would run several ten milers and half marathons, and employ my old training schedule leading up to November. I ran half marathons in Nashville, New Orleans, Baltimore, and Philadelphia. I ran an eighteen mile race on Long Beach Island in New Jersey three weeks prior to the marathon. I was strong and pain-free. I was ready!

Five years had passed since I last stood at the starting line of the New York City Marathon, but there I was, on Sunday, November 3rd, 2002 at 11:00am on the Verrazano Bridge, singing our national anthem, awaiting the blast of the starting cannon, and when it came . . . I took off with over 30,000 other like-minded runners with one a single goal in mind, crossing the finish line at Tavern on the Green in Central Park, 26.2 miles away.

I felt strong and I ran strong. I took it one mile at a time, remembering the course like it was yesterday—from the Verrazano Bridge, through Queens and Brooklyn, on to First Avenue, through the Bronx into Manhattan, turning up 58th Street and into Central Park. As I approached the finish line, tears filled my eyes. I knew I was back!

Chapter 2

Getting to know your bones

To understand osteoporosis, we must first understand our skeletal system, what it is, how it forms and equally important, how it ages. The way bones are formed and maintained is a complex process that involves environmental factors such as nutrition, sunlight exposure, and biological processes that involve various hormones, vitamins and minerals such as: the parathyroid and calcitonin hormones; vitamins D and K; calcium, phosphorus and other minerals.

HOW BONE FORMS

Bones start forming very early in the fetal life, grow significantly throughout child and adolescent development, up until age 18 to 21. However, the bones we are born with are not the same bones three years later, because we are really not born with bones. More on that later.

Every organ in the body, including the bones, goes through a process of building, destruction of the older parts and reconstruction. The bone cells that promote bone growth are called "Osteoblasts". The cells that reabsorb bone are called "Osteoclasts". As the body ages, the process of destruction is more active than the process of reconstruction which leads to progressive bone loss and the appearance of osteoporosis, unless we do something to balance the process, which brings me to exercise (not for the first, or last time).

Exercise is a primordial factor to maintain the bones' health. In fact it is found that women who are active as youngsters have the best bone mineral density at menopause. It is the action of gravity that stimulates the deposit of minerals in the bones, as long as these essential minerals are adequately ingested. Exercise is so critical that a person will lose up to 30% more bone mineral density after being in a cast for two months compared with the healthy limb. The matrix of the bone is sensitive to changes in the strain exerted on the bone during activity. Stress on the bone generates tiny electrical currents that attract calcium and other minerals to the site.

Bones are composed by 70% of mineral salts and 30% of an organic matrix formed primarily of collagen fibers, chondroitin sulphate and hyaluronic acid. The bones start forming when the osteoblasts produce the collagen and the ground substance formed by the chondroitin sulphate and the hyaluronic acid. Then, the various salts, especially calcium, start precipitating into this matrix to make it dense and strong.

Various calcium salts are the source of the most essential element in bone formation. Calcium in the blood is determined by the interplay between the absorption of calcium in the intestines, the excretion of calcium through the kidneys and its intake and release from the bones. All of these processes are regulated primarily by the above mentioned hormones. Other hormones, like thyroid, sex and stress hormones play a secondary role.

Calcium is a very important element not only in the structure of bones but also in the contraction of all muscles in the body, including the heart and smooth muscles of the blood vessels and the digestive tract, blood clotting; and nerve cell impulses. Too much of this important element will cause depression of the nervous system, decreased reflexes and slower electrical conduction in the heart; too little calcium will cause the nervous system to be excited.

Even with the influence calcium has over so many bodily functions, ninety eight point nine (98.9) percent of our calcium is stored in the bones and will be released from there into the compartment outside of the cells as needed. Only 1.1 % percent of the total calcium is inside the cells and in the blood stream. However, even a slight variation of calcium inside the cells will cause intense changes, with reactions like muscle contractions, even seizures. The body will take calcium out of the bones to maintain a stable level inside the cells and in the space between them. You can see now how a long term deficiency in calcium will cause loss of bone mass in order to maintain stable body function.

Calcium and Phosphorus

Calcium and phosphorus are closely related in the way they are managed. Eighty-five percent of the body's phosphorus is in the bones, about fifteen percent is in the cells, and less than one percent is in the space outside of the cells. Phosphorus also serves many important functions including the primordial energy management systems. Long term decreases of phosphorus will also cause loss of bone mass.

Bones can also be affected by other minerals like magnesium, sodium, potassium, copper, boron, and silica. The particular role and exact requirements of these micronutrients for proper bone health have not been exactly determined.

The usual intake of calcium and phosphorus is about 1,000 mg a day. This amount can be found in 2 cups of sea vegetables, 3 cups of collard greens or 4 cups of milk. Vitamin D is essential for the absorption of calcium; with it, the intestines absorb about 35% of the ingested calcium. Phosphates are absorbed readily and only the portion that combines with the non-absorbed calcium is excreted in the feces.

The kidneys also manage calcium and phosphate, however almost all of the calcium is reabsorbed. How much calcium is excreted depends on the concentration of calcium in the blood. Even a small increase of the calcium ion, the one that is not attached to proteins or in the form of a salt, will cause an increase of the secretion of calcium through the urine. The most important mechanism controlling the re-absorption of calcium is the parathyroid hormone.

The rate of elimination of phosphorus is directly proportional to the increase in the blood. Parathyroid hormone can greatly increase phosphate excretion in the kidneys.

Vitamin D

Vitamin D increases the absorption of calcium from the gastrointestinal tract, and has important effects on bone deposition and absorption. Vitamin D3 (Cholecalciferol) is formed in the skin by the action of ultraviolet rays on 7-dehydrocholesterol, which is formed in the body through enzyme reactions. Other forms of Vitamin D are absorbed from foods. Vitamin D and the converted forms are stored in the liver, from a few weeks to months.

The cholecalciferol gets converted to 25 hydroxycholecalciferol. The conversion of vitamin D is self-limiting; when the concentration rises beyond what is needed it will shut down the enzyme that makes it. The 25 hydroxycholecalciferol is converted into the most active product of vitamin D, the 1,25—hydroxycholecalciferol in the kidneys by the action of the parathyroid hormone (PTH). In the absence of the kidneys, vitamin D looses almost all of its effectiveness.

The conversion of vitamin D is inversely proportional to the concentration of calcium, the higher the level of calcium, the lower the rate of conversion. With a lower level of 1, 25 hydroxycholecalciferol there will be a lower rate of absorption of calcium from the intestines. Extreme quantities of vitamin D in the blood causes absorption of calcium from the bones.

Vitamin D is also important in the function of the muscles. In fact, supplementation of vitamin D and calcium in the elderly decreases the incidence of falls by 49% and improves muscle strength. It is necessary to administer calcium with the vitamin D to ensure its absorption.

Recent studies, including one conducted by Harvard University researchers discovered that most people have below optimal blood levels of vitamin D; and recommend that over half of the population supplement with 1,000 international units of vitamin D daily in order to achieve the lowest risk of bone fracture.

Parathyroid Hormone

The parathyroid hormone (PTH) is produced by four small glands located behind the thyroid gland at the base of the front of the neck. They are so small that at times surgeons may remove them unknowingly during surgery. This hormone promotes absorption of calcium and phosphates from the intestines by its action on the formation of active vitamin D, and re-absorption from the bones when the level of calcium in the blood drops. In the longer phase of action, the PTH stimulates the formation of osteoclasts, which reabsorbs calcium from the bones. This hormone also causes calcium to be re-absorbed in the kidneys, therefore preventing a total loss of calcium from the body. So, in general, PTH acts in absorbing and mobilizing calcium throughout the body.

Calcitonin

Calcitonin is secreted by the thyroid gland and it tends to decrease the concentration of calcium in the blood. In general it has the opposite effects of those of the parathyroid hormone (PTH). Its secretion is provoked by the increase in calcium concentration in the blood. It also inhibits bone re-absorption by its effect on osteoclasts. The effect of calcitonin is relatively weak in comparison to the action of PTH.

These are the main factors in the management of calcium, phosphorus and the metabolism of the bones. The interaction between them is very active. The amount of calcium absorbed into or lost from the body fluids is as much as 300 milligrams in one hour. The addition of this amount in one hour would be sufficient to cause serious hypo or hypocalcaemia (high calcium in the blood) with deadly consequences. The body has various buffer mechanisms to prevent this problem. The first line of defense is the deposit or removal of calcium and phosphate salts into and from the bone. About 5 percent of all blood circulates through the bone each minute, so about one half of any excess of calcium will be removed by this buffer in about 70 minutes. The second buffer is in the cellular mitochondria of various tissues in the body, the liver and the intestine primarily. They manage as much at 10 grams of the total amount of calcium in the body.

Vitamin K

Vitamin K is an important cofactor for the enzyme that activates osteocalcin. Osteocalcin is a protein produced by the osteoblasts, and is used within the bone as an integral part of the process of its formation. Vitamin K is also an important factor in the formation of matrix Gla-protein (MGP). MGP is synthesized in the smooth muscle cells of the healthy vessel wall and is a powerful inhibitor of calcification of arteries and cartilage, helping to prevent arteriosclerosis. It appears that optimal vitamin K levels are needed to produce proper amounts of MGP to prevent calcification and stiffening of arteries.

Vitamin K1 (phylloquinone or menaquinone 4) is found in dark green leafy vegetables. Vitamin K2 (menaquinone 7) is synthesized by intestinal bacteria, and is absorbed from the distal small bowel. Antibiotics have been shown to reduce vitamin K2 from this source.

Fermented foods typically have the highest concentration of vitamin K2. Natto is fermented soybeans eaten in Japan for over 1,000 years. It may be unpalatable for some people because of its slimy texture, but its vitamin K is far better absorbed than vitamin K from vegetables. Vitamin K2 blood concentrations after consuming natto have been shown to be about 10 times higher than those of vitamin K1 after eating spinach.

Japanese researchers found a statistically significant inverse correlation between the incidence of hip fractures in women and natto consumption. Even though fermented foods provide the highest source of vitamin K, a relatively low vitamin-K-containing vegetable like lettuce, eaten one or more times per day, has reduced the risk of hip fracture by 45% as compared to women who consumed lettuce one time per week or less.

Vitamin K has been compared to a first-generation biphosphonate drug (Didronel) in 72 osteoporotic women for two years. There was no significant difference found in the bone fracture rates between women taking vitamin K and those taking the biphosphonate drug for osteoporosis. Other studies have shown vitamin K to be equivalent to Fosamax-type osteoporosis drugs.

UNDERSTANDING OSTEOPOROSIS

Osteoporosis is a disease of the bones characterized by loss of bone mass and integrity of the bone architecture that leads to increased weakness of bones and risk for fracture. Interestingly, at the same degree of bone mineral density, an older person's bones are more fragile than a younger one's. This is because the strength of the bones is also determined by the collagen matrix that supports the structure of the bones. As we age, collagen in the body looses elasticity and integrity. Osteoporosis often goes undetected until a fracture occurs. The spine, hip, and wrist are the most common sites for fractures.

Osteoporosis is more common in women than cancer, stroke and heart disease combined. Primary osteoporosis is related to aging. By age 50, four out of ten women will have a bone fracture as a complication of osteoporosis. About half of postmenopausal women will have an osteoporosis-related fracture during their lives, including 25% who will develop a vertebral deformity and 15% who will suffer a hip fracture. This translates into over 1 million fractures annually in the United States. Many of these women will develop disabling chronic back pain.

Hip fractures are associated with a mortality rate of approximately 25% in individuals over 65 years of age. The other common site for fracture, the wrist, causes additional disability. Besides the pain and increased death risk people with osteoporosis may require long-term care and/or placement in a treatment facility due to limited ability to care for themselves.

Men also suffer from bone loss as they age. Two million American men have osteoporosis, (compared to at least 8 million women), and 3 million are on the verge of developing it. One third of all hip fractures occur in men. Bone loss in men usually occurs more slowly than in women and at later ages. By age 70, men will have lost one seventh of their bone mass. The bone loss in men does not usually produce symptoms until age 75 and older.

Chronic conditions, such as hyperthyroidism, renal disease, cancer, and hyperparathyroidism can accelerate bone loss and manifest secondary osteoporosis. If a secondary cause of osteoporosis is suspected, a laboratory assessment that includes a comprehensive thyroid and parathyroid hormone evaluation, calcium and vitamin D blood levels, complete blood count, metabolic panel, cortisol stimulation test, and erythrocyte sedimentation rate, need to be considered.

Why Women Are More At Risk

It is a known fact that as women age, go through menopause, and stop producing estrogen, it is natural to lose a certain amount of bone density. While this is a fact, it is also normal for women to pass through menopause and within eighteen months of completing menopause, have the same bone density that they had when they began the change of life process. So the stronger a woman's bones are when she begins menopause, the stronger they should be once menopause is completed. Unfortunately, as a result of poor dietary and lifestyle habits, many women are experiencing osteopenia (a pre-osteoporotic condition), and full-blown osteoporosis long before becoming pre-menopausal.

Normally thought of as a disease that affects postmenopausal women, today, everyone is at risk of developing osteoporosis and other bone related diseases at earlier and earlier ages.

Men Get Osteoporosis Too

A major cause of osteoporosis in men is elevation of the stress hormone cortisol which sucks calcium from the bones. In men, it is hastened by the inevitable downward drift of testosterone, which in turn starves bone tissue of its favorite hormone—estrogen. (Bone tissue uses a special enzyme, aromatase, to convert testosterone into estrogen.) Other factors, such as modern treatments for prostate cancer that block testosterone production to inhibit prostate cell growth, add to the pool of men at risk for osteoporosis and bone fractures.

Men over 50 are at a greater risk of osteoporosis-related fractures than they are of prostate cancer. Mortality in men one year after a hip fracture is twice that of women. Not only testosterone but also estrogen may be important in men's bone health.

The Risk to Our Children . . . Our Future

Our children consume on average of four soft drinks daily, two of those will contain caffeine. On top of this, there is the consumption of sugar, which also will affect bone density. As years go by, the bones will starve of the nutritional requirements to build a strong frame, during the most critical years of formation.

A 2003 study has linked regular cola consumption to lower bone mineral density (BMD). Among the subjects, regular cola drinkers had decreased BMD compared with infrequent drinkers. BMD was 2.3% lower in the trochanter, 3.3% lower in the femoral neck, and 5.1% lower in the Ward's area. The study showed that when phosphoric acid comes packaged with other nutrients, it is absorbed normally and everything is in balance. The problem with cola is that you are getting those doses of phosphoric acid without any calcium. It is not balanced, and that extra phosphorous bonds with calcium and prevents it from being absorbed.

THE DEMISE OF OUR BONES

The bones of people living in westernized countries are growing weaker. Women living several centuries ago had stronger bones. There is evidence that Near Eastern women had 20% higher bone mass twelve thousand years ago than women of today.

Some risk factors are unchangeable like: being female, Caucasian or Asian, aging, having a family history of osteoporosis and fractures, having prior fractures and medical conditions that may contribute to osteoporosis, such as thyroid or other hormonal disorders, and other medical conditions resistant to treatment, like Paget's disease.

Other factors can be changed, such as smoking, thinness (< 127 lb in women), early menopause (< 45 years of age, either natural or surgical), excessive alcohol intake (chronic alcohol use inhibits the function of the osteoblasts, the bone forming cells), a sedentary lifestyle (lack of weight bearing exercise), low calcium intake (women who diet frequently may limited their intake of calcium rich foods), poor general health and other factors. Neurological and ocular disorders may predispose to recurrent falls and increase the risk for fracture.

Medications

Long term use of corticosteroids, thyroid hormones, anticoagulants, tranquilizers like diazepam (valium) or lorazepam (Ativan) or anti-seizure medications also increases the risk for osteoporosis. All of these medications can affect bone metabolism negatively.

Diet

Dietary factors are extremely important. An imbalanced diet will predispose to a variety of disorders, not only osteoporosis. People go from one fad diet after another, most often to lose weight on a short term basis, rather than developing a lifestyle that incorporates healthy eating. Often, this will lead to long term health consequences. To much or too little of certain nutrients will predispose to a variety of conditions.

Caffeine Intake

Caffeinated coffee will induce excretion of calcium in the urine. Drinking more than 2 cups of coffee per day will lead to significant calcium loss over time, if you have a low calcium intake. It has been shown that coffee intake will increase the risk of hip fractures. (Hollingbery 1985; Heaney 1982, Hernandez-Avila 1991). However, green and black tea have been shown to help with bone mass buildup.

Alcohol

Alcohol intake has been linked to osteoporosis in males. About half of the men from 24 to 62 will suffer from osteoporosis. It is not yet certain if this is a result of a primary action of the alcohol or it is due to the poor nutrition that coexist with high alcohol intake.

Protein

The amount of protein ingested also increases the risk factor for osteoporosis. In a study, women with a high intake ratio of animal to vegetable protein had three times the rate of bone loss as compared with the group of women with a low ratio, and about four times the rate of hip fractures, even after adjusting for various factors including calcium and total protein intake. The digestion of animal protein unleashes large amounts of uric acid that the kidneys must excrete. Other studies have shown that when kidney function slows down with age and calcium intake drops, the body will use bone calcium to buffer the acid buildup consequently eroding the bone.

It is important to carefully assess the information received by the popular media regarding diet and nutrition. There is evidence that interest groups, such as the Milk Industry Foundation, disseminate scientifically unsubstantiated, probably deceptive and possibly harmful advertising about the need for milk as a staple in people's diet.

The idea that milk products are the primary source of calcium is false. In fact there is evidence that women who drink more than two glasses of milk daily have a higher risk of hip fracture than women who drink one glass of milk or less per week. In fact, women who drink extra milk show a negative calcium balance. The countries with the highest consumption of dairy products also have the highest rates of osteoporosis. In China, people's calcium intake is one half of the United States while their bone fracture is one fifth of that in the USA.

Sugar

The increased consumption of sugar in our diet has lead to an increase of the calorie intake in the form of simple carbohydrates, to the exclusion of other foods that could supply a richer content of other nutrients and minerals. Sugar depletes our bodies of calcium. Studies have suggested that sugar will mobilize the calcium from the bones and induce osteoporosis.

Increased sugar intake also increases the production of cortisol by the suprarenal gland. Even though this is a very important hormone, the excess production is just being under stress. Homocysteine is an amino acid produced inside the body as an intermediate product in the pathway towards other important biological compounds. An elevated homocysteine level appears to be a prominent and independent risk factor for osteoporotic fractures in older men and women. High levels of homocysteine are linked to heart disease and it also raises the risk of fractures even in people with a normal bone density level. Having high homocysteine levels doubles the chances of experiencing fractures.

The data was adjusted for age, gender, body mass index (BMI), smoking status and history of recent falls. The findings suggest that it is beneficial to use folic acid, cobalamin and pyridoxine to reverse high homocysteine levels.

Other Factors

Limit your intake of vitamin A, since it can weaken your bones. Studies have found that more than 6,600 IU of Vitamin A from food or supplements increases the risk of fractures in postmenopausal women. It also applies to men over 50: those with the highest blood levels of vitamin A had the greatest risk of fractures over a 30 year period. The main problem is supplements: don't take a separate Vitamin A pill, and your multivitamin should not contain more than 5,000 IU of Vitamin A, and at least 40% of it should be in the form of beta carotene. Beta carotene, a form of "vitamin A" is safe for your bones. Don't take cod liver oil and rarely eat liver which are the richest food sources of vitamin A. Check the labels on highly fortified breakfast cereals.

A history of absence of menstrual periods especially when associated with excessive exercise and/or anorexia nervosa will cause an imbalance in the main hormonal control center, the hypothalamic-pituitary axis, manifested by lower levels of estrogen, progesterone, and androgens that will favor osteoporosis. The intense physical overtraining will cause chronic stress that will impair mineral intake and absorption

Depression and stress are also risk factors because of the elevated cortisol level, a hormone produced in the suprarenal glands, and a consequent re-absorption of calcium from the bones.

Data shows that as the number of risk factors increase, for example: from 0 to 2, from 3 to 4, or more than 4, even at the same level of bone density, the risk of fracture increases.

Risk Factors in Osteoporosis

Unchangeable	Unmodifiable	Female Caucasian Asian Family History of Osteoporosis History of Fractures Paget's Disease
	Modifiable	Aging Early Menopause Thyroid Disorders
Changeable	Emotional	Stress Depression
	Habitual	Sedentary Life Physical Overtraining Eating Disorders (Anorexia Nervosa)
	Dietary	Tobacco Alcohol Coffee High Animal Protein Intake High Milk Consumption High Sugar Intake High Homocysteine Level High Vitamin "A" Intake Mineral and Vitamin nutritional deficiencies
	Medications	Thyroid Medication Antiseizure Medication Corticosteroids Anticoagulant Medication Tranquilizer Medication
	Heavy Metals	Cadmium

THE PROCESS OF AGING AND WHY DIET AND LIFESTYLE MATTERS

We have established the fact that we are all getting older, that we are not doing so very gracefully, that it seems to sneak up on us from out of nowhere, that osteoporosis is not just a disease that affects menopausal women . . . so, what next?. The key is our understanding and participation in the aging process. To better understand osteoporosis it is important to have some knowledge of how the body works and how it ages physiologically.

Understanding results in better judgment. Just taking a pharmaceutical because a doctor prescribes it is as extreme as running a marathon without training for it. We need to become active participants and understand the consequences of all of our actions and choices. When we become active participants in our health and well-being, as opposed to nervous spectators and unconscious followers, hoping for the best, it is then and only then we can truly begin the process of healing. Let's take a look at a simple model of how the body ages physiologically from the standpoint of our bones.

Our bones . . . our strong support system that literally allows us to stand is composed of living, moving tissue. Like all living tissue, our bones are constantly being built up and broken down. Healthy bones are the result of this process staying in balance . . . in step, if you will. When the breaking down of bone is equally matched by the building up of it, we feel strong and confident, secure that our skeletal structure is supporting us in every way.

How bones develop from just a few cells is, just like every other aspect of our miraculous bodies quite a miracle. In their infancy, bones start off as cartilage, a compound very similar to a very firm gel, eventually taking the shape of our future bones. Specialized cells in the shaft of the long bone start the actual bone formation growing toward the ends, while cells there also start to turn into bone.

Bones are comprised of a collagen matrix, which makes up about 35 percent of the bone, resulting in its flexible nature. In this matrix, calcium phosphate, a mineral salt is amassed, giving bones their strength. Seemingly rock hard, bones are constantly moving and changing, living tissue that replenishes itself as it wears down. From birth until sometime in our twenties, our bones build up much faster than we break down, resulting in growth and density. From our mid-twenties to about thirty years of age, we begin to see the change in the ratio of building versus breaking down. How that process continues in our bodies is largely dependent on how we eat, exercise, use pharmaceuticals and our overall health. Some bone loss, from 0.5 to 1.5 percent each year is normal and usually has no serious repercussions to our health.

How do we create a condition where our bones age gracefully and healthfully, staying strong? Is it all about calcium? Being hard and rich in calcium does not necessarily mean that our bones are not at risk of fracture. Bones can be dense and yet brittle, fracturing easily. It's important to remember that bones are a reservoir of numerous minerals essential to our health and function . . . calcium is only one. The most abundant mineral in the body, calcium is vital to our overall health and organ function, with our bones containing about ninety-nine percent of all the calcium in our body (the rest being distributed for use in everything from blood clotting to metabolism to hormonal function).

Balance in our bones, like everything else in life, is essential for their continued health. Too little calcium will result in deficient bone rebuilding, which means thinner bones. Too much calcium, on the other hand, can result in kidney and gallstones. Too little phosphorus can prevent the bones from making necessary calcium salts, weakening bones, while too much can stimulate the release of calcium from bones leaving them weak.

In addition to calcium, nutrients essential to bone formation and health include protein and vitamin C (to stimulate collagen matrix formation), vitamin D (to increase calcium absorption from small intestine to blood), magnesium (to increase calcium absorption into bone), exercise, strain (to increase the rebuilding of bone tissue), balance thyroid function (to slow bone loss). Other essential nutrients for bone health include boron, manganese, vitamin K, zinc, copper, silicon, vitamin B6 and folic acid.

Remember as well that we need to be aware of . . . and avoid, in my opinion, foods that weaken and drain our bones of their strength. As mentioned earlier, simple, refined carbohydrates like white flour and sugar, excessive caffeine, excessive alcohol, acid-producing foods like poor-quality vinegars, soda, low-fat and no-fat diets, over-the-counter antacids, excessive saturated fats and protein all contribute to bone loss and depletion by creating an overly acidic condition in our bodies.

As we age, we undergo a number of physiological changes which affect not only how we look, but how we function and respond to daily living. Overall, the changes we experience as we age involve a general slowing down of all organ systems due to a gradual decline in cellular activity. It is important to understand that we are all different, we have different genetic makeup, different life experiences, different ethnic backgrounds, different dietary and other lifestyle practices, all of which means we can experience these changes differently and at different times in our lives—for some, the aging process may be rapid and dramatic; for others, the changes are much less significant. While approximately 85% of older adults experience chronic conditions, only about 20% experience significant impairment in their ability to function.

We don't know yet all the causes of aging but one thing we know is that as we age, the cells in the body do not function as well. We know that the accumulation of waste products from oxidation processes and free radical damage decreases the function of various organs, and all the hormone systems slow down in function. Which is why the primordial hormone, or metabolic dysfunction, driving the process of aging has not been determined. Decrease in Growth Hormone is a significant factor. This hormone is critical in the stimulation of new cell growth and repair of tissue damage.

Some people propose that the deficiency of melatonin is the basic mechanism through which aging changes occur. Whether this hypothesis is true or not, the fact is that melatonin levels drop with age and the use of melatonin is beneficial in aging.

The Outward Signs of Aging

The most common external signs of aging involve our skin, hair, nails, and overall stature. Over time, our skin loses underlying fat layers and oil glands, causing wrinkles and reduced elasticity. Our hair gradually loses its pigmentation and turns gray. Our nails become thicker due to reduced blood flow to the connective tissues. Our overall stature changes as our muscles atrophy and our bones lose density and compress.

While aging is inevitable, how we do it is largely the result of a lifetime of eating and lifestyle habits. How we age has a dramatic impact on our bones from many standpoints.

Changes in Musculature

A generalized atrophying of all of our muscles is normal in later years accompanied by a replacement of some muscle tissue by fat deposits. This results in some loss of muscle tone and strength. Some specific implications are reduced ability to breathe deeply; reduced gastrointestinal activity which can lead to constipation; and bladder incontinence, particularly in women. Although everyone experiences these changes to some degree, regular physical exercise appears to temper the extent of these changes. Toned muscles, strong muscles take some of the burden off our aging skeleton.

Changes in the Skeletal System

Beginning at around age 35 in both men and women, calcium is lost and bones become less dense. This can result in osteoporosis and a reduction of weight bearing capacity, leading to the possibility of spontaneous fracture. Thinning of our vertebrae also results in a reduction in height. In addition, the vertebrae calcify, resulting in postural changes and increasing rigidity, making bending difficult. Our joints also undergo changes. In fact, arthritis, the degenerative inflammation of the joints, is the most common chronic condition in the elderly. The two most common forms are osteoarthritis, a wearing away of the joint cartilage, and rheumatoid arthritis, a disease of the connective tissue. These conditions can impair mobility and our performance of regular daily activities.

Changes in the Nervous System

After age 25, everyone loses nerve cells. Gradually over time, this results in a reduced efficiency of nerve transmission, affecting response time and coordination. Our brain also shrinks in size, which does not significantly affect functioning except in the most extreme cases. These changes may also affect our sleeping patterns somewhat by decreasing the length of total sleep time and REM sleep. However, new research has shown that there can be new cell growth even in the aged and that is why it is so important to remain active both mentally and physically to prevent the development of dementia. Now we know that old dogs can learn new tricks.

Changes in the Gastrointestinal System

As we age, we experience a reduction in the production of hydrochloric acid, digestive enzymes, and saliva, as well as a reduction in the total number of taste buds. These changes can result in gastrointestinal distress, impaired swallowing, and delayed emptying of the stomach. Perhaps more important, the breakdown and absorption of foods may also be impaired, sometimes resulting in vitamin deficiencies of B, C, and K vitamins or, in extreme cases, malnutrition. If left untreated, these deficiencies may result in capillary weakening, easy bruising, muscle cramping, reduced appetite, weakness, mental confusion and/or illness, and of course bone loss.

Changes in the Endocrine System

Our endocrine system is responsible for changing food into energy and coordination of metabolic functions. After age 25, everyone experiences approximately a 1% decrease per year in their metabolic rate. This overall slowing results in food being less efficiently absorbed and utilized, as well as a decrease in our overall metabolism of drugs. Consequences can include bone loss, reduced stamina and reserves as well as greater susceptibility to drug toxicity.

It's never too late to change

How we maintain our muscles . . . with exercise; how we eat and digest impacts the health of our bones; our metabolic functions directly impact our bones; both when we are young and as we age. The more information you have about how your body works and how it ages can directly impact the density of your bones.

Before you jump into the casket know that how you live your life has a profound affect on how you age. So many times people tell me, "oh, it's too late for me." I'm here to tell you 'IT'S NEVER TOO LATE TO CHANGE'! There have been countless numbers of studies that show the positive effects of both diet and exercise, both physical and mental, on aging at any age. Recent studies show people in their eighties and nineties seeing profound changes within days of beginning a moderate exercise program, so, it's never too late to change.

DIAGNOSING AND RECOGNIZING SYMPTOMS OF OSTEOPOROSIS

Primary osteoporosis, as noted earlier, is related to the aging process. Older women are at a higher risk of fractures partially because of the increased risk for falling due to other medical conditions.

In evaluating the risk for osteoporosis and fractures it is important to identify the changeable risk factors, including the general health, weight (as was noted above in risk factors, low body weight can promote osteoporosis), and Bone Mineral Density (BMD). Often the first sign of osteoporosis is a broken bone, but loss of bone density can be detected before the condition worsens. And you can take action.

DEXA Scan

There are a number of methods that measure bone density, including: dual-energy x-ray absorptiometry (DEXA); single-energy x-ray absorptiometry; quantitative CT; and quantitative ultrasonography of the heel.

The DEXA scan is the most frequently used and most studied method. Its reliability has been validated and is, we could say, the "gold standard" for assessing the BMD. The test is usually covered by insurance companies to be performed every two years after age 65, or in women who are at risk or have developed osteoporosis at an earlier age due to other factors, like an early menopause.

Bone Mineral Density

There can be differences in the Bone Mineral Density in different areas of the body at the same time, such as the wrists, the hip, lumbar spine, forearm or the heel. One area may be more or less affected in the same person at one time. The areas of most concern are the hip and the spine.

DEXA scan reports can be difficult to read. They provide both a "T-score" and a "Z-score". The T-score is the number of standard deviations above or below the mean (more or less the average) BMD for sex—and race-matched young adults. Standard deviations are the "outliers" within the same sex and race population. The Z-score compares the patient with a population matched for sex and race as well as age within 1, (one), standard deviation below mean peak bone mass.

The World Health Organization (WHO) suggests that osteoporosis is present when the bone mineral density (BMD) is 2.5 standard deviations or more below the mean for healthy young adult women at the spine, hip, or wrist (corresponding to a T-score lower than or equal to—2.5). Osteopenia (decreased bone mineral density) is defined by a T-score between-1.0 to—2.5; a normal T-score is—1.0 and higher. The categories of osteopenia and osteoporosis were established because fracture risk is not a threshold. It's a gradient risk. The risk increased progressively from one diagnosis to the other. There are people in the osteopenic category that, particularly if they have additional risk factors, may fracture. It's important to recognize that those in the osteopenic group are also at risk for fracture even though the highest risk may be seen in the patients with osteoporosis.

Most experts agree that all women should have their BMD measured by age 65 and that early treatment will prevent the risk of fractures. Some suggest evaluating women at risk (i.e.: low weight, early menopause, family history, prolonged hormone replacement therapy, etc.) at around age 60. Men aged 70 years and older and anyone with a fracture occurring after a disproportionate cause like falling from a standing height or lower, and those with possible secondary osteoporosis should also be evaluated for bone density. Additional testing may be required to monitor treatment.

Bone Resorption Assessment

As the bones break down, not only is calcium removed and put in circulation, but there are also residues of the breakdown of the collagen matrix of the bones. The Bone Resorption Assessment test focuses on two collagen crosslinks with great specificity for bone resorption: pyridinium (Pyd) and deoxypyridinium (D-Pyd). These compounds are measured in urine. The presence in urine of higher than normal amounts of Pyd and D-Pyd indicate a rapid rate of bone loss. A high rate of bone turnover in an untreated postmenopausal woman indicates that bone loss is likely to be rapid.

Nearly all women will show high bone turnover in the first few years after menopause, but about one third will continue to have high turnover ten to twenty years after menopause. Many clinicians believe such women are destined to suffer extensive bone loss and should be targeted for aggressive therapy to block bone resorption. Women with fractures and osteoporosis excrete higher levels of collagen crosslinks into the urine.

Patients with recent fractures show higher excretion of both markers than those without recent fractures, indicating that accidental bone fractures also increase crosslink excretion. The test can also help to determine the efficacy of treatment without having to take a DEXA scan every four to six months.

PREVENTION: YOUR FIRST CHOICE

The best preventive strategy is to decrease all the modifiable risk factors. Therefore, it is imperative to encourage the development of a healthy lifestyle that includes proper nutrition, an adequate exercise program and control of other risk factors for osteoporosis, including encouragement to stop smoking and avoidance of excessive use of alcohol.

Management of stress is indispensable to promote excellent health and to prevent not only osteoporosis, but other preventable medical conditions. Meditation and relaxation techniques, prayer are helpful to reduce the stress hormones. Learning proper breathing techniques also helps to manage stress. I often suggest audio programs such as: "Breathing: The Master Key to Healing", and "Meditations", by Andrew Weil, MD.

There are several centers in the body where the autonomic nervous system has a concentration of ganglions and nerves. It is probable that each of these centers influences particular emotional states, and these in turn affect specific organ systems. These centers appear to correspond to what the Indian yogis call the chakras. According to theory, to address the emotional issues that influence osteoporosis, it is critical to address issues of dependence versus independence, capability versus fearfulness, and trust versus mistrust.

The center involved in the predisposition to osteoporosis is the first one, located at the base of the spine. It is related to issues with family of origin, with physical safety and security in the world, and the sense of belonging. A healthy emotional first center function will manifest with strong sense of self and power which will permit a sense of independence, resourcefulness, fearlessness and the ability to trust. Disturbances associated with this center can manifest as an excess of power, with rejection of support or help from others, and possibly recklessness. You can also see the development of unreasonable trustfulness which can be naive. Each of the seven centers has connections to various emotional states and organic functions.

If there is much to deal with and process emotionally, individual counseling or psychotherapy will be necessary. There are various schools of psychotherapy. Commonly found schools are the psychodynamic, the cognitive-behavioral, interpersonal, humanistic, gestalt, bioenergetic, etc. If you decide you need help dealing with emotional conflicts and unresolved issues, make sure you find a practitioner who is warm, caring, understanding and supportive. Also, it is preferable that the therapist is eclectic, able to integrate various styles and strategies that may apply to your issues. Even though research has shown that all therapies produce favorable and similar outcomes, particular therapies may be more adequate in dealing with particular issues.

Three to four sessions are sufficient for you to determine if a practitioner is right for you. Within that time a practitioner should be able to present a cohesive treatment plan and prove an understanding of your situation. You should feel comfortable and understood. Don't hold back on shopping for the right therapist if you don't feel these standards are met. The greater your mental and emotional wellbeing and integration the better your organism will respond to biological interventions.

Often, nutritional and mineral supplements will be necessary at times to provide necessary elements to fight disease. These supplements will be discussed in chapter 3.

Ways for the elderly to prevent fractures include fall prevention strategies by safety-proofing the home by removing loose rugs, installing safety bars in bathrooms, and using night lights. Canes and walkers should be encouraged for those with gait disturbances.

Research also shows that hip protectors, which look almost like bicycle shorts, may reduce fractures by 50%. The only limitation to this approach is that many women do not want to see themselves with larger hips.

It is also important to discuss with your primary doctor all of the prescriptions and over-the-counter medications that may cause lightheadedness or interfere with balance. Finally, regular eye examinations to ensure adequate vision with updated eyeglass prescriptions can help decrease the risk for falls.

If you are treated with medications that can potentially affect bone metabolism, discuss with your doctor, or with other consultants, the possibility of decreasing or even stopping the medications. Make sure you do not change the dosage or stop the medications you are taking without consulting with a physician experienced in the conditions you are suffering from and in the management of the medications you are taking.

Ultimately, prevention should always be your first choice. You and you alone have the power to make that decision. You can take control over your own destiny and do everything possible to maintain and/or regain your health, or you can choose to accept the consequences that come with living an unhealthy lifestyle. And it is never too late to start. And there is no such thing as, "it's too late for me". Begin where you are and don't look back. The choice is yours.

Part 2

The Path to Recovery

Chapter 3

Treating Osteoporosis

WHAT I DID

Armed with my diagnosis, I began a serious evaluation of my overall health and the choices I made over my life that led to my current condition. It's very easy when facing a major health crisis to retreat and become depressed. A very positive person by nature, I was determined to figure out the "why" and "how" of my condition, realizing that my diagnosis didn't mean that I had "gotten" osteoporosis out of the blue, but rather it had been developing for quite some time. The only thing that had changed was my newfound awareness.

There is a certain amount of responsibility that comes along with a major health concern, one that will involve making life-changing decisions. The way I see it, you can accept your diagnosis, fill your doctor's prescription, take pharmaceuticals, change nothing else in your life, and hope and pray for the best outcome. Or, you can go on a quest, as I did, to discover the root cause of your condition, realizing you only begin the healing process once you understand the cause. Here's where the responsibility part comes into play . . . big time.

My Approach

I had to unconditionally accept the fact that I chose osteoporosis. No, I didn't wake one day and say, "I think I want osteoporosis." I did, however, make life choices that had a profound effect on my condition. Yes, there was a lot to take into consideration other than those choices: heredity; environmental issues; lifestyle; etc. As I did, you will need to establish a starting point, and that starting point should always be the effect your own free choice had on creating the situation you find yourself in.

I had to understand, too, the complexity of my situation. Many people, armed with a health crisis, look for a quick fix: a magic pill, a surgical procedure, an experimental protocol; when in reality, there is never a quick fix. Osteoporosis is a complex condition of a major organ system, in many instances caused by years and years of inappropriate dietary habits and a lack of physical activity. If you have it, you've probably had it for quite some time, and it is not going to go away in a month, or even a year. And opting for taking the most commonly prescribed pharmaceuticals will, in most instances, only increase your bone density by one to three percent over the course of a year. My point is, no matter what path you choose to take, conventional medical procedures, alternative therapies, or a combination of both, it's going to take time, patience, discipline and determination. Don't expect you'll begin any program and see a difference in a week or a month, but, know that time goes by, and time can heal all. Provided you take an active role.

The following are the steps I took . . . and strongly recommend you consider on your path to building strong healthy bones.

I found a doctor who would be a partner and take a pro-active role in my journey back to health

This is an extremely important. While it is imperative that we accept responsibility for creating our conditions, and while it is equally important that we take an active role in our own health, we need doctors. I am not a medical basher. I needed, however, to find and work with a doctor that I could trust and who would include me in all the decisions pertaining to my health. I needed to be an active partner in my recovery. I needed a doctor who was expert at creating health. I needed an expert in alternative medicine since that was the path I was choosing to take for my treatment. I chose Dr. Merizalde for all those reasons and more.

Also, if you suspect you have a medical problem, don't wait. If you have a symptom or symptoms that persist, rather than self-medicate, over supplement or make an assumption you know what it is, get a definitive diagnosis; then decide what to do about it. When I suspected that something was seriously amiss, I went for help. Sure, I was surprised by my diagnosis, but I needed to know.

Just as I did, when dealing with a health concern, find a doctor who you like and trust, who will work with you, especially if you choose to research an alternative approach to healing. Ideally you will search out and find a medical professional with a leaning toward alternative health, one who will revert to conventional therapies only if deemed absolutely necessary.

Today it is becoming easier and easier to find such a medical professional; however, it's easy to understand why so many modern doctors are reluctant to look at alternative approaches to healing. First and foremost, many alternative approaches are completely untested. There is no scientific proof that they work.

Secondly, everyone today is a self-proclaimed health expert claiming to have the latest cure for whatever ails you. With so much information, it is important to work with a medical professional who can be helpful in guiding you in an appropriate direction.

I reviewed and modified my diet

I put a lot of emphasis on diet because I believe it is the leading cause of osteoporosis in our culture today. My own shocking diagnosis was osteoporosis caused by malnutrition; and at the time, I ate what I believed to be an extremely healthy diet; a diet based on whole grains, fruits and vegetables, minimizing excessive fat and protein. And while minimizing saturated fat is a good thing and always will be, in my research, I learned so much about fat, protein, and other nutrients important to creating and maintaining optimum health

Christina decided that we needed to start with a clean slate. She convinced me that we had to throw out everything we knew and re-visit how we thought about food and how it affects us day to day, using what we knew to create a new way of eating. The very food I thought had nourished me for all these years had become the root cause of my current crisis. I will admit that I came to many of the changes she was recommending kicking and screaming. After all, I ate a 'perfect diet,' as healthy as diets come, and had done so for thirty years. Everything she was recommending was everything I had eschewed for all those years. I was scared and Christina knew that feeling, so she gently nurtured me along, allowing me to get comfortable with each change, while at the same time, making sure the changes were made so I could regain my health.

In my years of practicing a strict macrobiotic approach to eating, my diet consisted primarily of whole grains, in particular brown rice, as well as beans, tofu, tempeh, lots and lots of vegetables, cooked in a variety of ways, sea vegetables, nuts, seeds, a small amount of fruit and an even smaller amount of fat, and no animal protein to speak of.

Now, my purpose here is not to denigrate the macrobiotic approach to healing; but I now understand that the austere approach that Christina and I took to eating was perfectly suited to her healing, but not perfectly suited to keeping us nourished as we lived healthy and very active lives. There were just not enough calories, not enough fat, not enough protein . . . not enough nutrition . . . period! So it was time to alter how we looked at food.

What we did

The first change we made was a tough one for me. Christina thought that we needed to cut back on my volume of whole grains. We would continue to eat them every day, but we cut back on the volume. I was a little worried, as I was always hungry and wondered if I would get enough to keep me going, especially now. Which brings me to the second change . . . the amount of fat and protein we consumed.

All our research showed that I was, in truth, starving, although I made very healthy food choices. Without enough fat in my diet, many of the nutrients I took in were not being properly assimilated. So I was not benefiting, leaving me constantly hungry. We increased my intake of fat, through the use of olive, avocado, and flax and hempseed oils, a wide variety of nuts and seeds, including flax and hempseeds, and foods like avocados which we generally avoided in the past. When I say increased, I mean increased.

Prior to making these changes, we sautéed vegetables with a tiny bit of oil once or twice in a week's time. Now, we were sautéing every day, several times a day, with liberal amounts of oil. We made salad dressings, sauces and toppings, all with extra virgin olive oil or avocado oil as an ingredient. We added flax and hempseeds and flax and hempseed oil, a tablespoon of each per day, to increase my intake of the essential fatty acids, specifically omega-3, much needed for cell renewal, an imperative need for my condition.

And then there's salt. That most precious ingredient that keeps our blood strong and mineralized, when consumed in balance. When eaten in excess, however, it can wreak havoc with your health . . . in particular your bones. While we used only the best quality of salt, soy sauce and miso, as well as sea vegetables for our health, we used far too much of these ingredients, contributing yet again to the demise of my bones. We continued to cook with salt, but with a much lighter touch. We reduced the frequency with which we served sea vegetables, but kept them in our repertoire of foods since they are so mineral rich.

I knew that protein was important for strength, but I did not think we needed a lot of it. I quickly changed my mind as Christina increased our intake of all kinds of protein: tofu: tempeh: beans: and for me, fish. I had not eaten fish in years, except on the rare occasion. Eating it, along with more beans, soyfoods and fat changed everything for me. I was stunned at how quickly I gained wait, going from a mere 128 pounds to a hearty 148 pounds. Plus, I felt stronger, more balanced and had more energy.

These changes were dramatic for me, but in truth, all Christina did was enhance and improve on our already healthy diet. The changes we made re-established my foundation so I could rebuild my health and my bones.

A side note on how we eat

We like to think we are an extremely well-informed culture, when it comes to diet and nutrition. We count calories; we're obsessed by fat grams and carbohydrates; we're conscious of every morsel we put into our mouths, but when you get right down to it, what do we really know about diet and nutrition, and how do we actually apply it to our daily lives? What's a macronutrient versus a micronutrient? Have you ever actually seen a carbohydrate or fat gram, and if so what did it look like? How important is calcium . . . really . . . in preventing osteoporosis?

And what about fat and protein and phytonutrients? Confused? Know one thing; every time you open your mouth and put something into it, from that eye-opening cup of coffee in the morning to your bedtime snack, it impacts the health of your bones.

As a culture we don't really cook very much anymore; cooking has become just another chore to endure at the end of the day, if we do it at all, and food has become the enemy. As a result, we eat prepared foods, restaurant food, take-out food, fast food, microwaved food, food out of cans, freezers, boil bags and boxes, foods laced with chemicals and pesticides.

We don't eat very much that is truly fresh and alive. Food that is fresh has life force and energy; it nourishes us quite differently than food out of a can, box or package. When we consume a meal prepared in this manner, we feel nourished and satisfied. Our dietary practices are in need of a major overhaul. Our bones are our deepest organ system, and like all of our organ systems they require proper nutrition in order to maintain optimal health and strength in order to carry us through our lives.

It is imperative, if faced with a diagnosis of osteoporosis, that you review and modify your diet. I recommend searching out a center for integrative medicine that employs medical professionals and nutritional counselors who embrace modern thinking when it comes to diet and nutrition. And always remember, it's your body; take control; understand what's going on; ask questions, and then ask more questions. If something isn't resonating with you . . . don't do it! Nobody knows your body better than you.

In chapter 6, 'Diet for Healthy Bones,' we cover dietary influences on bones in great detail, including: facts about fats and oils, good fats versus bad fats; the effects of simple carbohydrates such as refined grain and sugar on the health of our bones; we'll discuss the role soy products, flax and hemp foods, and other proteins play in building strong healthy bones; and we'll look at the havoc caused by dairy products, caffeine, alcohol, colas and carbonated beverages, and excessive sodium. And if that's not enough, in Part 3, 'The Diet Connection,' we provide you with one hundred and fifty mouth-watering recipes for healthy bones created by Christina.

I implemented an osteoporosis supplement program

Working with Dr. Merizalde, we developed what we believed to be the ideal supplementation program for osteoporosis. What follows is a list of suggested supplements. In chapter four, "Treating Osteoporosis for Life," we have included a complete explanation of each of these supplements and how they work in the body to aid in the prevention and cure of osteoporosis.

Supplement	Dosage	Frequency
Calcium Complex for Bones	400 mg	3X daily
Magnesium	1000 mg	3X daily
Vitamin D-3	1000 intl units	2X daily
Liquid Silica	1 tablespoons	1X daily
Glucosamine and Chondroitin	1000/750 mg	3X daily
MSM	2000 mg	3X daily
Red Yeast Rice	200 mg	2X daily
SAMe	200 mg	2X daily
Vitamin C	1,000 mg	3X daily
Zinc	50 mg	1X daily
B Complex	50 mg	1X daily
Melatonin	0.5 mg	1X daily
Flax or Hempseeds	1 tablespoon	2X daily
Flax or Hempseed oil	1 tablespoon	2X daily

I worked with a physical therapist and implemented a weight-bearing exercise program

As an athlete, no one had to convince me that exercise would play a leading role in helping me to regain my bone health. I also understood that if I planned to run again, I had to listen to the experts and work my body out in a way that could support its healing. In each of the physical therapy sessions I took, I worked as the therapist directed and followed their expert advice. Working with my physical therapist helped reduce my pain, increased my strength and helped me remain active.

My experience is that most conventional doctors will own up to the importance of weight-bearing exercise in treating osteoporosis, but they will do so in a very conservative manner. In many instances, you'll be advised not to take on an aggressive exercise program for fear that you will break a bone, fracture a hip, experience multiple stress fractures, etc. That is where a good physical therapist comes in.

If diet is the leading cause of osteoporosis in our culture, then lack of physical activity and weight-bearing exercise is only second to it. Bottom line, regardless of your age, I believe you need to do weight bearing exercise, you need to build up to the point where you are doing it vigorously and aggressively, and you must make it part of your daily routine. It is what I did, under the supervision of my physical therapist and a certified personal trainer. That doesn't mean put down this book this instant and run to the gym and start lifting hundred pound dumbbells. That would be irresponsible and extremely dangerous as well.

Numerous studies have shown that regardless of age, or at what point in your life you begin a physical exercise program, everything from weightlifting to running to yoga and kick boxing can have a profound effect on your overall health, both physically and psychologically.

I recommend requesting a prescription from your doctor for physical therapy. In most instances, physical therapy is covered by your health insurance. At first your doctor may question the importance of physical therapy and may ask why you think you need it. Insist on it. (Most osteoporosis doctors will just want you take a prescription medication and have an annual DEXA scan. The doctor who originally diagnosed my osteoporosis questioned me when I inquired about physical therapy.) With prescription in hand, you need to search out and find a physical therapist specializing in working with athletes and sports related injuries.

While some physical therapy clinics can be very depressing, it has been my experience that those specializing in helping athletes get back to their sport are the exception. You will find extremely motivated patients who want to get back to their daily routines as quickly as possible, as well as supportive, encouraging therapists who want to help them get there. It will be a very positive experience.

Your physical therapist must understand your condition, and the importance of building your core muscle groups, along with the ligaments, tendons and connective tissue that support them. Understand that if your bones are osteoporotic, then your muscles are most likely atrophying and your tendons, ligaments and connective tissue are contracting. This should be his or her primary concern. Your core muscles are the largest muscle groups in your body. They are the muscle groups that support your lumbar spine (lower back) and hips, the areas of the body most affected by osteoporosis.

Once your core muscles are sufficiently strengthened, your next task is to find a personal trainer. Your physical therapist can most likely refer you to someone, and while this will not be covered by your health insurance, it will be money well spent. Like physical therapy, you don't want just any personal trainer, but rather a responsible certified exercise physiologist who can design and monitor an appropriate weight bearing exercise program for your condition, age, and body type.

The rest is up to you. You need to be committed, determined, positive, disciplined, and diligent. It is therefore important that you seek out professionals who will work closely with you to identify and develop a program that not only resonates with you, but one that you will enjoy doing. No matter your age, if you don't enjoy doing something, the benefits you receive from it, while helpful, will not be as profound as they would be if you were to embrace it with great joy and anticipation.

A final thought on this step. My own experience is that adopting an exercise program, while difficult at first because you are not used to doing it, changes everything about your life. When you exercise aerobically, endorphin levels are elevated in the brain. Endorphins can be described as morphine-like substances manufactured in the brain during exercise. The net result is exercise can become a positive addiction. So while you are working at becoming stronger and healthier, you may also find that you feel better about yourself; have a more positive attitude; handle stress (a major cause of osteoporosis) better; become more emotionally stable, more confident, and more self-sufficient. So instead of feeling depressed and bad for yourself, lace up those athletic shoes and give it a go!

I researched both conventional and alternative treatments and therapies

For many people, the easiest approach to illness is a visit to the doctor, fill the prescription and attempt to get on with life, hoping for the best. I am not saying that there is never a place for medical intervention or a need for prescription medications. That was not for me. I believe very strongly that I, the patient, had to take an active role in understanding my condition, and work to achieve optimal health. It is my body; I live in it and I, who really and truly knows what's going on inside. And I had to understand that I . . . and only I . . . could fix it. So I researched all of my options first . . . and took nothing as the 'only way' or the 'absolute truth' until I had all the facts. I did my homework so I could make an informed decision.

My experience and suggestion is that you employ the experience of three different modalities regardless of your condition. In this instance, since we are talking about osteoporosis, you need to see an osteoporosis specialist in order to get a clear and concise diagnosis of your condition, and the severity of it. This way you will know what you are dealing with, as well as get a good picture of what conventional therapies are available to you. Now you've got a place to begin your research.

Secondly, you need to search out and find a medical professional who can work with you on an alternative approach to your condition. This doctor can review all of your tests and recommended therapies, and determine if an alternative approach is appropriate. He can also speak to your osteoporosis doctor on your behalf, in medical terms, regarding any alternative approaches you decide to follow. More research . . .

Thirdly, find a nutritional counselor, preferably one who has studied traditional Chinese medicine, who can work with you on implementing a dietary program specifically for your needs. One designed to build your bone density. Sorry, more research. It is then and only then that you can make an informed decision.

I took all three of these steps. I saw an osteoporosis doctor at a major hospital. I left his office with a prescription for Fosamax, and a referral to a rheumatologist and a nutritionist. I immediately began my search for a second opinion and used an alternative approach prior to following the recommended conventional route and taking any prescription medications. I also worked with my wife, Christina, a student of Chinese medicine and nutrition expert, and together we reevaluated my diet, and made appropriate changes taking building bone density into consideration.

I did a ton of research, and the results speak for themselves. Today, having annual DEXA scans in order to track my progress, doctors have seen an unprecedented improvement in my bones.

I kept a positive attitude and outlook toward life with an emphasis on doing the best I knew how each and every day

There is a song that begins "Life's a dance you learn as you go; sometimes you lead; sometimes you follow."

I realized early into my recovery that all I could do was wake-up each and every day; get dressed; nourish myself the best way I knew how. I put the needs of others before my own; tried to be kind to everyone I encountered, and got on with my life. In my opinion it is really that simple. Accept life without condition, and know that you chose the hand you were dealt. Not happy with it? Change it. And when you run head-on into what may seem to be a devastating catastrophe, (or when one runs into you), which is bound to happen, remember, it's just life. It happens to everybody. And if you need professional help dealing with it, that's fine too. Get it.

We've all heard the sayings, 'don't be attached to the outcome,' and 'no matter where you go, there you are'. One of my favorites is not so well known, 'to believe in you is more than I need to make believing more than making believe.' Putting the needs of others before your own, keeping a positive attitude, and doing the best you know how each and every day makes all the difference in the world, especially when you are dealing with a health crisis. It changes everything. You'll find yourself smiling and laughing more; you'll attract more positive energy; you'll experience everything differently. And most important, you'll discover the difference between finding a cure for your condition and truly healing.

Realty Check

There are 3 goals of osteoporosis management:

1)   stop or reverse bone loss;
2)   increase or stabilize bone mass; and
3)   reduce fractures, pain, disability and mortality.

If you have medical conditions that can contribute to unhealthy bones, make sure you educate yourself about what you suffer from and what alternative approaches could help. Know about the various treatments available and discuss your findings with your doctor in order to sort out the validity of the information. There are many books and websites that can offer good ideas; many others will be rubbish and have no substantiation. Your doctor should be able to discuss your findings with respect and understanding, as discussed earlier. I can never stress enough how important this relationship is to your recovery.

As we have already discussed, exercise, diet, and control of other changeable risk factors is essential for the management of low bone density and osteoporosis. After that, there are other particular supplements and compounds that are significant in the prevention and treatment of osteoporosis. Many of the approaches from a nutritional or supplementary nature are no longer considered alternative. Many of these supplements are supported by scientific studies and are now part of conventional medicine.

Chapter 4

Treating Osteoporosis for Life

NON-PHARMACOLOGICAL TREATMENTS

Diet

I could rant all day about the importance of understanding your dietary needs and food choices in the recovery of your bone health. I have discussed my own choices and how I modified my healthy approach to eating to support my own recovery.

Many people who suffer with osteoporosis, do so as a result of poor dietary choices and misinformation as a result of marketing. It seems that dieting is a national pastime, and has been for many decades. If you believe everything you see on bookshelves today, you'd think carbohydrates are the root of all nutritional evil. Go back twenty, thirty, forty years and fat was the culprit. Bottom line is we need good quality fat and protein, and we need complex carbohydrates too.

A little culinary history for you, some of the factors for such a huge increase in osteoporosis today actually go back thirty and forty years when major changes in our dietary practices and food production began to take hold, and when the baby boomers of today where in their 20's and 30's. The first dietary changes had to do with food processing, the use of chemicals in our food, higher annual consumption of saturated fat, sugar, caffeine, soda, and consumption of more processed foods. These practices eventually lead to the fast food movement and a time when Americans consumed more meals out of the home . . . meals that were not properly balanced and therefore less nutritious.

Later, so-called advances in food production included the use of growth hormones in dairy and meat production. Dairy cows and beef cattle were no longer fed their natural diet of grass, but were rather fed grain, not a natural source of food for them. This unnatural diet led to the development of stomach, esophageal and digestive diseases in animals requiring the use of antibiotics. Growth hormones used in food production, causing faster maturation of animals, have been linked to early puberty in both girls and boys, which can result in lower bone density and eventual osteoporosis. Antibiotics in food production have been linked to antibiotic resistance in humans. Today's soda-gulping youth will suffer even more serious osteoporosis than we see today, even before they reach mid-life, as a result of excessive sugar consumption.

In the 70's and early 80's, as women got fatter, and the incidence of heart disease in both men and women increased, we identified the enemy . . . dietary fat. Rather than attack the real enemy, saturated fat from over consumption of animal protein, we attacked all fat, and the low-fat, no-fat diet approach was born. For the next twenty to thirty years, it seemed everything we ate, to the detriment of our health, which needs dietary fat to assimilate fat soluble nutrients, was no-fat or low-fat.

Today we have elevated our food production to a whole new level of insanity with more chemicals used in agriculture and food production than in any other industry. And these same chemical companies that have infiltrated our food chain over the last half century, have now created the biotech era and the creation of genetically modified food.

While there is a complete section in this book on diet and recipes for healthy bones, it is important to note here to make certain you follow a well balanced diet, educate yourself on food, avoid fad diet crazes, and get adequate amounts of protein, healthy fats and complex carbohydrates. Include at least 5 servings of vegetables daily, especially those green leafy vegetables. Ideally eat seven to nine servings of a variety of vegetables and fruit per day, with the emphasis more on vegetables and less on fruit because of its high sugar content. One serving is about one ounce. Even if you decide to follow a balanced vegetarian or vegan diet, you will have as many of the necessary nutrients as you will need.

The daily recommendations for protein has ranged from 0.5 to 1 gram of protein per kilogram of weight (1 kg = 2 lbs, roughly). According to calculations, an adequate diet should contain at least 10% of the calorie intake in the form of protein. Most vegetables, grains and nuts have at least this percentage of protein. Meats have between 45% and 68% of their calories in the form of protein. Brown rice has 8% of its calories in the form of protein; barley has 11%; pumpkin seeds 21%; lentils 29%; mushrooms 38%; tofu 43%; collard greens 43%; spinach 53%; and watercress 78%. As we mentioned previously, it is important to maintain the amount of animal protein at the lower level to prevent loss of bone and increase longevity. Animal protein, especially dairy products, also tend to cause more allergies.

Because of the close relationship between female hormones and bone health it is important to improve the perimenopausal status by following a program of exercise, diet, herbal and nutritional supplements. Phytoestrogens, isoflavones, are the most important compounds to balance female hormones. Phytoestrogens are present in soy and flaxseed, in red leaf clover and kudzu root. Some women will need hormone therapy to manage menopausal symptoms and/or osteoporosis. Later in this book you will find other supplements you may consider helpful.

The healthy fats include the omega-3 fatty acid linolenic acid, which is found in seeds, particularly pumpkin, flax, hemp and sunflower; and the omega 6, linoleic acid which is found in grains and vegetable oils. All other fatty acids are derived from these two. DHA, found in breast milk, is essential for the proper development and function of the brain. However, it is not produced in a significant amount until two years of age. Eicosapentanoic Acid (EPA) and Docohexaenoic acid (DHA) are also found in fish. These fatty acids, the omega-3, produce compounds from the series 1 and 3 of the eicosanoids, which are anti-inflammatory compounds.

The usual dosage of omega-3 and 6 fatty acid required is 3-6 grams per day. This dosage can be found in 2 tablespoons of flax or hemp seed. The advantage of hemp seed is that it has a more ideal proportion of 1:4 between the omega-3 and omega-6 fatty acids.

Trans-fatty acids are the most dangerous fats for health. They can be found as part of many processed foods and are called hydrogenated fats and oils. They are produced commercially because they extend the shelf life of commercial food products. However, they contribute to the production of compounds in the body called eicosanoids, which are mediators of inflammation. Inflammation is a contributor to cancer, heart disease and osteoporosis.

Saturated fats are found in animal products, mollusks and shell fish. They also contribute to heart disease and inflammation. The most wide spread fatty acid in this category is Arachidonic acid, an omega 6 fatty acid. Because meat has a higher percentage of calories in the form of fat, it is a major contributor to obesity. In animals that are grass feed, and are free roaming, there is a higher level of omega 3 fatty acids, which are anti-inflammatory therefore, balancing a bit the presence of arachidonic acid.

Essential fatty acids are required for the structure of every cell in the body, making them essential to bone health.

Nutritional Supplements

I was always of the belief that dietary supplementation with vitamins, minerals and herbal remedies was unnecessary provided one got plenty of exercise and ate a well balanced whole foods diet with plenty of whole grains, vegetables, soups and stews; while avoiding processed foods, simple sugars, dairy and most animal food.

It seemed to me that pill popping had become a national pastime . . . all kinds of pills for all kinds of reasons. Prior to my diagnosis, I never took supplements or pills of any kind for that matter, but armed with my new found information, and a prescription for the popular osteoporosis drug Fosamax, one of the areas I decided to research, prior to filling the prescription, was vitamin, mineral and herbal supplementation. My research was eye-opening to say the least. I discovered that supplements had gone way beyond taking vitamin C to prevent a cold.

Osteoporosis Supplementation

It is very important to note when it comes to supplementation, we are all very different, and we all have very different nutritional needs. This is a very complex issue, even though the vitamin manufacturers, like pharmaceutical manufacturers would want you to believe otherwise. So many factors go into determining our individual nutritional requirements at different phases of our lives, which is why it is important to note that when dealing with any medical condition, it is imperative that you work with a medical professional prior to just adding supplementation to your daily regimen.

While many supplements can be harmless, studies have shown that based on a person's condition and prescription drug medications they may be taking; and we take a lot of them in this day and age, supplementation can sometimes have an adverse affect when combined with prescription medications. I worked closely with Dr. Merizalde, and based on my DEXA scans, MRIs, blood work, lifestyle, family history and other factors, we decided to hold off on filling the Fosamax prescription and instead developed an appropriate program combining homeopathy, supplementation, and follow-up testing.

The first supplement that comes to mind when you think about bones is calcium, so I began my search there.

Calcium

While calcium is the most abundant mineral in the body, with about 99 percent of it deposited in our bones, one would think that calcium should be a first defense in the fight against osteoporosis. And while it is true that numerous studies have shown high levels, between 1000 and 1500 mg a day, of calcium supplementation can help reduce bone loss by between 30 and 50 percent, other studies have shown that there is no link between osteoporosis and calcium depletion.

Preventing osteoporosis isn't as simple as taking a calcium supplement. The reality is that bone tissue is complex, dynamic and alive, and like other tissue in the body requires a wide range of nutritional needs. Prior to just adding calcium supplementation, one may want to consider having a blood and urinalysis testing to determine if in fact calcium absorption and depletion are an issue. Remember, everyone is different.

If calcium is an issue for you, you need to understand that the form in which you take a calcium supplement is crucial. Calcium supplements come in various forms such as: citrate, aspirate or carbonate formulation, amongst others. The citrate form is best absorbed on an empty stomach while the carbonate preparations should be taken with meals. While calcium carbonate may have the highest percentage of elemental calcium, it is the most poorly absorbed at about 4 percent, while calcium citrate has an absorption rate of nearly 50 percent. And be wary of calcium supplements derived from bone meal and dolomite as they have a high lead content, (a known toxin), and are also poorly absorbed by the body. Antacids with added calcium are not good choices for calcium supplementation, because antacids will decrease chlorhydric acid which is necessary for optimum calcium absorption. Besides, they contain no magnesium, which is necessary for optimum bone health.

Postmenopausal women are recommended to take 1500 mg daily of calcium supplementation; those who are taking hormone therapy are advised to take 1 g per day. Iron supplements and thyroid medications decrease the absorption of calcium and should be taken at a different time of the day than calcium. Vitamin D will improve the absorption of calcium.

Large doses of calcium can also result in a magnesium deficiency; therefore, if you take large doses of calcium you need to make certain that you increase your intake of magnesium. Most calcium supplements designed and sold for bone support take this into consideration and include magnesium at a ratio of 2 mg calcium to 1 mg of magnesium. In some situations you may require a higher amount of magnesium, for example, if you suffer from asthma, cramps and high blood pressure. Another reason why it is important to discuss supplementation with your doctor.

Ensuring adequate dietary calcium intake can be difficult if you don't consume a significant amount of food rich in calcium. Supplementation is advisable for people whose dietary intake is inadequate.

Also, as discussed earlier, don't assume if you drink milk and eat dairy products that you are doing your bones good. There are vegetables that have higher rates of calcium absorption than milk, even if milk has a higher concentration of calcium. Only 32 % of milk's calcium is absorbable, while 63.8% of the calcium in Brussels sprouts is absorbed. Other foods that have higher calcium absorption rates than milk are: mustard greens, broccoli, turnip greens, and kale. You can get the same amount of calcium in a glass of milk as in a ½ a cup of firm calcium-enriched tofu, 1.5 cups of broccoli or 1/3 cup of sesame seeds.

Vitamin D

Vitamin D is also a major factor when taking a calcium supplement. Vitamin D is one of the most important regulators of calcium. It enhances calcium absorption in the intestines and decreases the excretion of it in the kidneys. We need vitamin D to maintain the body's blood level of calcium in the appropriate ranges to maintain essential cellular functions and to promote bone mineralization.

Until recently, the recommended daily allowance of vitamin D was four hundred international units. This was the amount required for adequate calcium absorption. Recent studies; however, indicate that amount should be increased to a minimum of 1000 international units daily, to as much s 2000 international units.

The most natural source of vitamin D is spending time outdoors in the sun. Something we don't do as much of as we used to. Even our children spend more time indoors today staring at computer and television screens. In addition to supplementation, being outdoors in the sun is still one of the best ways to get vitamin D. Playing, exercising, walking outdoors is our best source of this crucial vitamin. Fifteen minutes of sunlight per day on the face and forearms generate adequate amounts of vitamin D; however, the sun's rays above 45° latitude are too weak in winter to generate the proper amount of vitamin D production.

Individuals in geographic regions where the sun is not strong enough for vitamin D production, and institutionalized individuals who do not receive daily sun exposure, will probably require vitamin D supplementation. It is important to note that vitamin D is not effective on its own; it requires the presence of calcium and dietary fats for the proper absorption, not only of Vitamin D but also A, E and K. If taking vitamin D in supplement form, be certain to take it with a fatty meal.

It is also important to determine the level of vitamin D in blood to assess the adequacy of the intake and/or supplementation. There are two vitamin D tests—1,25(OH)D and 25(OH)D. The correct test is 25(OH) D, also called 25-hydroxyvitamin D. Normal 25-hydroxyvitamin D lab values are: 20-56 ng/ml or150-140 nmol/l. Your vitamin D level should never be below 32 ng/ml. Any levels below 20 ng/ml are considered serious deficiency states and will increase your risk of breast and prostate cancer and autoimmune diseases like MS and rheumatoid arthritis. The optimal 25-hydroxyvitamin D values are: 45-50 ng/ml or 115-128 nmol/l.

Magnesium, Boron, Zinc, Manganese, Copper

These are all important nutrients in maintaining the health of our bones. Other important minerals whose role is not completely clear are required at the following dosages: magnesium, 600-800 mg; boron, 4-12 mg; zinc, 15-50 mg; manganese, 2-5 mg; copper 2-3 mg. These minerals are often found in multivitamin complexes and calcium and bone support supplements.

Vitamin K

Vitamin K is one of the most important nutritional interventions for improving bone density. It serves as the biological glue that helps plug calcium into bone matrix. A number of studies indicate that women who suffer from osteoporosis and bone fractures have 35% deficiency of vitamin K, increasing the risk of bone fractures six-fold.

The minimum daily dosage necessary is 70-140 mcg. The best sources of vitamin K are leafy green vegetables. Eggs have some as well. The best sources of vitamin K are: collard greens (400 mcg/100g), spinach (380 mcg/100g), salad greens (315 mcg/100g), kale (270 mcg/100g), broccoli (180 mcg/100g), Brussels sprouts (177 mcg/100g), and cabbage (145mcg/100g).

For treating osteoporosis, some oral forms of Vitamin K have 500 mcg per drop, so 6 drops would give the recommended 3000 mcg per day, the amount found in over one pound of collard greens. Collard greens or spinach will be enough for preventive purposes but if you already have osteoporosis, or heart disease, extra vitamin K will assure that your bones will be healthier and your blood vessels won't harden.

Unlike vitamin D, which is toxic in large doses, vitamin K1 (phylloquinone) is not toxic at 500 times the RDA. However, synthetic vitamin K3 (menadione) toxicity has occurred in infants given vitamin K3 by injection.

Vitamin K requires at least an ounce of fat to optimize absorption, so, it is important to have a diet that includes sufficient essential fatty acids. The same goes for the other fat soluble vitamins A, D and E. Supplemental vitamin K1 may be six times more available than vitamin K1 in a food source like spinach

CAUTION: If you are taking the blood thinner Coumadin you need to use vitamin K with caution because it will reverse the effects of this medication. You may still take the vitamin K under the supervision of your physician, but you should first have your PT (coagulation) and Coumadin levels measured and the dosage readjusted to compensate for the vitamin K effect. Vitamin K does not cause increased blood clotting: it only normalizes clotting. You could overdose on natural (not synthetic) vitamin K without negative effects on blood clotting.

Silica

Researching silica, I found this trace mineral to be important for the proper growth and maintenance of skin, hair, nails, ligaments, tendons and bone. The most obvious outward signs that silica is effective is noticeable improvement in both the hair and finger and toenails.

It also made sense to me that if my bones were osteoporotic, then most likely my muscle was atrophying and my tendons and ligaments were contracting and tightening. So silica seemed to be an appropriate mineral supplement to add to my daily routine.

Further research showed that silica is required for the formation of collagen in bone, cartilage, and other connective tissue. It is also essential for the normal skeletal growth by playing a role in the initial stages of bone development when the protein matrix is constructed. The human fetus has an abundant supply of silica in its unborn tissue in order to accomplish this. Some studies have shown that silica may also increase the rate of bone mineralization as we age, and that it plays a role in the formation of apatite crystal, the primary constituent in bone.

WOW! Pretty interesting stuff this silica, so what is it and why hadn't I heard more about it? Though silica-containing herbal plants, most notably horsetail, have been known for a long time in folk medicine, silica's restorative powers have been ignored by the medical establishment. Yet a hundred years ago the great scientist and healer. Dr. Louis Pasteur, proclaimed silica the ultimate future remedy. Silica puts calcium back into the bones and provides the major lubricant in our bodies. Nature provides silica, a vital nutrient, in a number of whole unprocessed foods. It is especially plentiful in whole oats and other whole cereal grains. Yet, through the over-refining and processing of grains and the continuous and combined onslaught of impeding environmental pollution, bad eating habits, and loss of adequate absorption ability, i.e., aging, body silica diminishes with age. To get it back into the tissues, we can boost silica metabolism though supplementation.

Glucosamine, Chondroitin and MSM

Supporting the health and proper function of our joints is crucial as we age, and when dealing with osteoporosis. Joint pain affects everybody at some point in time, and it is perhaps the most debilitating form of pain. Life is very different when you are unable to get in and out of a chair or a car, or worse yet, unable to get out of bed. Inability to climb up or down steps, or to reach up to get something out of a cabinet, or the simple act of opening a jar can prove devastating. I experienced all of this with my diagnosis of osteoporosis and the numerous joint related stress fractures I suffered.

As discussed throughout this book, one of the first defenses in both preventing and battling osteoporosis is to get sufficient weight bearing exercise, brisk walking, jogging, weight lifting, etc. By building muscle through weight bearing exercise, our bones become stronger; however, in the process of performing weight bearing exercise, our joints take a beating, especially as we age, so it is very important that you pay attention to the health of your joints, and do everything to prevent them from drying up and becoming stiff and painful, thus preventing you from exercising. Most people hate the thought of exercise to begin with; joint pain is the ultimate excuse not to do it.

As we have seen, silica can be a major aid in the health of our joints, but my research lead me to other supplements as well. Because I was experiencing extreme joint and back pain most of the time, Dr. Merizalde suggested I supplement with MSM, and in the process, I discovered glucosamine sulfate and chondroitin for joint health as well.

Let's begin with a look at MSM. MSM was isolated by Robert Herschler and Dr, Stanley Jacob of the University of Oregon Medical School in the early 1980's. Their research revealed that MSM, or methylsulfonylmethane, is a natural sulfur compound found in all living organisms, including human body fluids and tissue. It is actually one of the most prominent compounds found in the human body, just behind water and sodium. A 160 pound man has approximately 4 pounds of sulfur as body weight.

MSM is created in the atmosphere's ozone layer when sulphide is oxidized by UV light to form MSM (methylsulphonylmethane) and DMSO (dimethylsulphoxide) which itself then transforms into MSM. (Commercially MSM is made by burning DMSO.) The MSM create in the upper atmosphere, falls to the ground in the rain and is absorbed by plants through their roots.

MSM is our prime source of bio-available sulfur which is lost from our food by processing, drying, cooking and preserving. MSM is an important nutrient and is a component of over 150 compounds. It is needed by the body for healthy connective tissue and joint function, proper enzyme activity and hormone balance, along with proper function of the immune system. Research studies have shown that MSM is helpful in improving joint flexibility, reducing stiffness and swelling, improving circulation and cell vitality, reducing pain and scar tissue, and breaking up calcium deposits. It also has been shown to act as an analgesic and anti-inflammatory, and inhibits muscle spasm and increases blood flow, thus relieving chronic joint pain in many instances.

MSM is not a vitamin or a drug. It is an odorless, water-soluble, white crystalline material that supplies a bio-available form of dietary sulfur; it is non-allergenic, and has no interfering or undesirable pharmacological effects. Approximately half of the total body sulfur is concentrated in the body's muscle, skin and bones. Sulfur is necessary for making collagen, the primary constituent of cartilage and connective tissue. It is important to note, that studies suggest that the level of MSM in the body, like many other compounds, decreases with aging

Moving on to glucosamine and chondroitin: glucosamine is a combination of an amino acid, glutamine and a sugar, (glucose). It is concentrated in joint cartilage where it is incorporated in longer chains known as glycosaminogylcans (GAGs), and finally into very large structures known as proteoglycans, (chondroitin), whose function it is to attract water into the joint space for lubrication of the cartilage during movement in order to maintain structure and repair damage. Studies also suggest that glucosamine and chondroitin supplementation may also stimulate cartilage cells and begin the production of new healthy cartilage matrix. Other benefits include quickening recovery from connective tissue injuries, reduced joint pain, increased joint lubrication and anti-inflammation of joints.

Glucosamine has been shown to be as effective as non-steroidal anti-inflammatory drugs (NSAIDS), such as ibuprofen, without any known side affects. It has also been shown that, whereas the effects of NSAIDS tend to wear off quickly, the effects of glucosamine last much longer, and slow the progression of symptoms. Research suggests that continued supplementation (1500 mg glucosamine and 750 mg chondroitin daily), can not only prevent joint structure changes, but it is believed it can also regenerate healthy new cartilage. As well, the decline in glucosamine sulfate synthesis with age may imply that a prudent anti-aging strategy may be to use a low-to-moderate dose supplementation as a prevention strategy beginning at 45 to 50 years of age.

Many glucosamine supplements also contain added chondroitin. Research suggests a ratio of two parts glucosamine to one part chondroitin for best absorption. Some experts question whether chondroitin can be absorbed, and suggest your body should make all the chondroitin it needs from the glucosamine it produces or the supplements you are taking; however, there may be a small group of people who don't produce enough of the enzyme required to make chondroitin from glucosamine. These are the people who benefit from taking it, but with no known side affects, I would recommend supplementing with both glucosamine and chondroitin.

You can find glucosamine and chondrotin, along with MSM in pill, powder or liquid form. You may want to consider a liquid or powder form versus pill, for better absorption and assimilation.

Red Yeast Rice

Of the supplements I take as a part of my daily osteoporosis regimen, red yeast rice is probably the most controversial; but in my opinion, perhaps one of the most effective in restoring the health of my bones. As noted earlier, I was doing osteoporosis research on line in November 2001 when I found a link to a study on osteoporosis and red yeast rice. The research indicated that supplementing with red yeast rice could result in a substantial increase in bone density in as little as twelve to sixteen weeks.

Again, I asked myself what is this stuff, and if it could increase bone density in people with osteoporosis in as little as sixteen weeks, why hadn't I heard about it? This lead me to do more research. The first and most important discovery I made was that not all strains of red yeast rice are the same. I learned that red yeast rice contains many different phytochemicals that have a variety of health benefits. These include many kinds of isoflavones and monacolins. Several of these phytochemicals are bone active. Also, due to variations in the process of fermenting the yeast on the rice, there are variations in the phytochemical content, which result in different levels of bone activity for different strains.

Some strains of red yeast rice are not bone active at all; therefore, it is important that I relate the brand name of the product I use since in my research, it is the only one to date that I have found that makes the claim to be bone active. This claim is certified by International Bone Laboratories (IBL). IBL consists of a group of scientists who are qualified to verify the anabolic effects on bone of small molecule compounds. IBL was organized in response to the demand from manufacturers and marketers of bone-related health products who wanted to demonstrate that their products are bone active. The product I use is marketed under the brand name OsteoSun which is distributed by Cell Tech, Klamath Falls, OR. (For more information, and to order this product call 1-800-939-3909.)

Red yeast rice is white rice fermented by a strain of red yeast called Monascus Purpureus. Native to China, it has been used in Oriental food preparation since 800 A.D. It is the red border on Chinese spareribs, it is used to make a type of red sake, and it is used for coloring other Asian foods. It has been discovered that this fermented food contains a compound called mevinolin, which is identical to the prescription drug, lovastatin—prescribed to lower cholesterol. Lovastatin is a prescription drug that comes with many warnings, therefore I do not recommend you supplement with red yeast rice for any purpose without first talking to your doctor, and observing the many warnings and cautions that come with supplementation.

While supplementation is important, red yeast rice is an excellent illustration of why we must not take the consumption of dietary supplements lightly, and of how the discovery of natural medicines can work in reverse. We are accustomed to discovering natural compounds within plants that are known to have certain properties or effects on the body, extracting them, and using them as medicines. Here, we have the development of a drug in a laboratory that is later discovered to be identical to a compound in a natural state in a food, and now being used for its effect on the body. (Note, however, that the monacolin in OsteoSun is 10 to 50 times less than the related statin amount in the statin drugs.)

Red yeast rice should not be combined with any other cholesterol or lipid-lowering drugs. It should not be taken if you have, or are at risk for, liver disease or have a history of liver disease. You should not take it if you have undergone organ transplant surgery. It should never be taken with grapefruit juice. Grapefruit juice can cause a buildup of lovastatin in your body, which can be dangerous. It should also not be taken with high doses of niacin.

So how does red yeast rice regenerate bone tissue? Certain strains of red yeast rice contain monacolins (phytochemicals) that activate the promoter of the bone morphogenetic protein 2 (BMP) gene. Osteoblasts are cells that are responsible for bone growth. Osteoblasts differentiation is enhanced by BMP-2. The monacolins in OsteoSun were identified from a library of 30,000 natural compounds as the most anabolic. Human bone cells exposed to these monacolins show enhanced expression of BMP-2 messenger RNA. When tested in a living body, these monacolins showed increased bone formation of 2—to 3-fold.

My personal experience was profound. I began taking the OsteoSun brand of red yeast rice in November 2001. I had my next DEXA scan sixteen weeks later in March of 2002. That DEXA scan showed an unprecedented increase in my overall bone density of over 9% in my hips and nearly 7% in my spine. Equally important to note, I had been suffering on-going recurring stress fractures for three years. Since supplementing with red yeast rice I have not experienced a single stress fracture.

SAMe

S-Adenosylmethionine (SAMe) is a naturally occurring compound that is involved in many biochemical processes in the body. SAMe plays a role in the immune system, maintains cell membranes, and helps produce and break down brain chemicals such as serotonin, melatonin, and dopamine as well as vitamin B12. SAMe also participates in the making of genetic material, known as DNA, and cartilage.

Most often used for mild depression, liver disorders, and joint health, numerous scientific studies indicate that SAMe may also be useful in the treatment of fibromyalgia, Parkinson's disease, migraine headaches, Sjogrens disorder (which causes pain in connective tissue), attention deficit/hyperactivity disorder in adults, vascular disorders, and even Alzheimer's disease (studies suggest that people with Alzheimer's disease have low levels of SAMe in the brain and that supplementation can actually increase those levels).

I began supplementing with SAMe for two reasons, first to relieve the sudden state of depression I found myself in as a result of my staggering diagnosis and not being able to run. You have to understand that running was not something I did for exercise or to pass the time. Running was, (and is) who I am. I am first a runner; everything else follows. Anybody diagnosed with a serious medical condition will not doubt experience some depression; it's only natural. SAMe is a safe, nonaddictive alternative to prescription medications. Secondly I took it for joint health. I believe you can not do enough to support the health of your joints.

If you decide to supplement with SAMe, start with a low dose (for example, 200 mg per day), and increase slowly if needed, as recommended doses vary depending on the health condition being treated. It is important to note that SAMe is extremely unstable and must be manufactured and packaged in a very specific environment. It is very susceptible to humidity. Look for enteric-coated tablets and make certain the packaging clearly states "Full Potency".

Vitamin C

No longer just to prevent the common cold, vitamin C is just beginning to be recognized as a major player in bone health. A 1997 study published in the Journal of Epidemiology and Community Health compared the difference between dietary and supplemental vitamin C. The study showed that postmenopausal women who took supplemental vitamin C for more than ten years had a higher bone density level than women who did not take any vitamin C. Interestingly, the study further demonstrated that frequent intake of foods rich in vitamin C was not associated with increased bone density. The study concluded that dietary vitamin C does not seem to be associated with bone health, but supplementation does.

If you choose to supplement with vitamin C, best to start with 500 to 1000 mg daily as calcium ascorbate (buffered form).

Zinc

Scattered throughout the body you will find approximately 2 grams of zinc. The highest concentration is found in the prostate, eyes, liver, and bone tissue. Zinc is an important factor in preventing osteoporosis. Zinc regulates the secretion of calcitonin from the thyroid gland and influences bone turnover. Maintaining adequate levels of zinc is important in traditional treatment of osteoporosis.

If you choose to supplement with zinc, take 30 to 60 mg a day in its most absorbable, chelated form: zinc glycinate, zinc picolinate, and zinc citrate. Also note, the absorption of zinc, like calcium, can be inhibited by certain foods, including legumes, whole grain cereals and breads, wheat bran, and brown rice. For maximum absorption, take your zinc at a different meal.

Essential Fatty Acids

Probably the most misunderstood of the food categories is fat. Fat is an essential part of a well-rounded and healthy diet . . . the body needs fat. Fat is required for energy production and to supply essential fatty acids and aid in the absorption of fat-soluble vitamins, (A, D, E, and K). Avoiding all foods that contain fat reduces the variety of foods eaten and can lead to nutritional deficiencies. My diagnosis of osteoporosis was linked primarily to malnutrition. My diet was severely lacking in fat and protein. My body was not assimilating important nutrients that it needed to metabolize strong healthy bone. My idea of cooking with oil was brushing the sauté pan with a teaspoon of oil once, maybe twice a week. And my concept of protein was eat all the bean and bean products I could find.

Adding a substantial amount of good quality fat and oil to my diet was the beginning of my turnaround. In six months time, changing nothing more than adding fish and fat to my existing diet, (which was extremely high in whole grains, beans and bean products, veggies, and sea veggies), I went from an unhealthy looking 128 pounds to a hearty 148 pounds. This was weight that my bodied needed.

The major components of fat are short chain molecules known as fatty acids. All fatty acids are classified according to their carbon-hydrogen makeup into three categories; saturated, monosaturated and polyunsaturated. The human body is capable of recognizing and utilizing all of theses types of fatty acids, but for optimum health, 60 to 80% of the intake should be polyunsaturated fatty acids.

Specifically, there are twenty different types of fatty acids that the human body needs for optimum health. It can manufacture all but two of them. These two are the Essential Fatty Acids (EFAs) omega-6 linoleic acid and omega-3 linolenic acid. These are termed essential, because they cannot be made in the human body and must be supplied by diet. If you consume whole grains, nuts and seeds, and fresh cold water fish caught in the wild, (not farm raised), several times weekly, you are most likely getting sufficient essential fatty acids in your diet. If not, you may want to consider supplementing.

I recommend adding hemp seed, hempseed oil and hemp protein powder to your daily diet as opposed to supplementing with pills or flaxseed products. For optimum health, the World Health Organization recommends that omega-6 and omega-3 EFAs be consumed at a specific ration of 4:1. The ratio of omega-3 to omega-6 in hemp products is 3.75:1. In flaxseed products it is 1:4, the exact opposite to the recommended 4:1. No other fat or oil on the planet comes close to as perfect a ratio of omega-3 to omega-6 as does hempseed.

Ipriflavones

Eat your tofu and drink your soymilk. Compounds like Genistein and Daidzein are from the family of the isoflavones. Soy is the main source of ipriflavones, which are responsible for many of the positive effects of soy in the body including the decrease of mood swings, PMS symptoms, migraine headaches, irregular periods, weight gain by decreasing fat and increasing lean tissue in menopausal women, decrease of the risk of breast and cancer, and the decrease of calcium loss through the kidneys. There are some reports that soy may decrease thyroid function, but other research has proven that there is no connection between the use of isoflavones from soy and thyroid disease. These benefits have not been found in the isolated isoflavones however an artificial isoflovone called ipriflavone has been found to increase bone density.

Two to three small servings of soy will provide about 40 to 60 mg of soy protein per day. This is the amount determined to be sufficient to have a noticeable clinical effect. It may take up to twelve weeks to see an effect on menopausal symptoms like heat flushes. Most women will need about 100 to 160 mg per day to have relief of menopausal symptoms like heat flushes, vaginal dryness and to protect their hearts and bones.

B Vitamins and Folic Acid

Research has shown that high levels of the amino acid homocysteine is linked to fractures in people who have osteoporosis. One way to keep your homocysteine levels in the healthy range is to take a vitamin B complex.

Food sources enriched naturally with vitamin B and calcium include broccoli and green leafy vegetables, carrots, avocados, cantaloupes, apricots, almonds, peanuts, nuts, and enriched foods. In patients with an existing deficiency or limited intake of foods rich with folic acid, or with a high homocysteine level, 400 to 800 mcg of folic acid per day is necessary. It is important to make sure that there is no deficiency of vitamin B12, because folic acid may mask the neurological problems that may occur from the lack of B12.

Melatonin

Melatonin is a hormone produced primarily during the night by the pineal gland which is located in the center of the brain and derived from serotonin, an important modulating neurotransmitter. Melatonin is very important in the regulation of sleep (the day-night cycle) and mood, and may have other important roles in the modulation of the immune system including the control of cancer cells, breast, colon and prostate cancer in particular. It has also been found to have powerful antioxidant effects and may have neuroprotective effects in patients with amyotrophic lateral sclerosis and Alzheimer's

The action of melatonin may vary depending on the dosage. In general, the lower dosages (0.5 mg) have a more physiological activity than the higher dosages (5-20 mg). At these lower dosages melatonin helps to regulate the adrenal glands and stress hormones.

Melatonin has been found to regulate calcium metabolism by stimulating the activity of the parathyroid glands and inhibiting both calcitonin release and prostaglandin synthesis. A decline in melatonin may be an important contributing factor in the development of postmenopausal osteoporosis. One investigator has even suggested using oral doses of melatonin combined with light therapy for prophylaxis and treatment of post-menopausal osteoporosis.

There are still a lot of unanswered questions regarding melatonin especially around the particular effects from different dosages. Research has shown that the results of a trial can depend on the dosage, the immune status of the individual, the pineal gland's status, the presence of stress and the circadian rhythm of the immune system. Therefore, the use of melatonin should be done with caution in people suffering from asthma, autoimmune conditions and adrenal insufficiency.

A Comprehensive Melatonin Profile test is a non-invasive analysis of melatonin in saliva over the complete light-dark cycle. This test may show melatonin imbalances that may play an important role in the development and progression of osteoporosis.

The usual starting dosage is of 0.5 mg, and according to the results of a saliva test to measure the levels, and the clinical response, the dosage can be increased. Usually it is not necessary to use more than 10 mg, however, some practitioners have used up to 50 mg. The quality of the various compounds available in the market is variable so at times it is difficult to know if you are getting the melatonin advertised in the bottle.

Melatonin may cause, rarely, minor adverse effects such as headache, drowsiness, insomnia, rash, upset stomach, or nightmares. The side effects occur especially at the higher dosages. The compound has extremely low toxicity; however, as noted elsewhere, caution has to be exercised in patients suffering from asthma, autoimmune or adrenal gland disorders. Caution also needs to be exerted in patients undergoing cancer chemotherapy since melatonin can affect tumor growth depending on the time in which it is administered. If melatonin is used in the morning it may stimulate tumor growth, if used in the evening, which is usually the case, it will slow down tumor growth. Melatonin may also exacerbate bipolar disorder and classic depression.

The bottom line on supplementation

Our research convinced us that supplementation in our fast food culture shouldn't even be a question; it should be a requirement. And even if we eat the most perfect healthy diet, we are all getting older. Science is learning so much about the human body, the aging process, the effects of environmental pollution, and so much more, that to not supplement in order to keep our immune systems functioning, our hearts pumping, our joints limber, and our bones dense is ludicrous at best.

THE ROLE OF EXERCISE

The subject of exercise and osteoporosis is an extremely important discussion. It could be the subject of an entire book. Since everyone is different, I do not intend to recommend various types of exercise, except to say that in the both battle and prevention of osteoporosis, it is imperative that you make some form of weight bearing exercise a major component of your daily routine, regardless of your age or condition.

If you are suffering with osteoporosis, you can take all the pharmaceuticals and supplements in the world, but without regular weight bearing exercise, you will struggle to gain substantial and adequate bone mineral density.

There is no excuse for not exercising. Everyone can do something, and you have to start somewhere. It is important that you take on an activity that is appropriate to your condition at the time you begin, and that you progress from that point. It would be wise to talk to your osteoporosis doctor, and get his input on seeking the advice of a professional physical therapist, as well as a sports medicine doctor, a physiatrist, who can assess your condition, recommend an appropriate program, and monitor your progress.

You will want to incorporate simple stretching and yoga type exercises, as well as meditation as part of your routine. This, in conjunction with weight bearing exercise, from lifting light weights to brisk walking, dancing, light jogging to all out running several days a week, will be the most beneficial means by which to prevent osteoporosis as well as to build strong dense bone.

Physical activity is clearly indispensable not just because of its positive influence on bone mass but also because it improves balance and strength and will prevent falls. The positive effect of resistance exercise on osteoporosis is well established. Researchers have found positive correlations between lean body mass and bone mineral density, meaning that the more active a person has been throughout life and the more muscle mass instead of fat, the healthier the bone mineral density. It was found that total body weight is not correlated with healthy bones therefore obesity will not promote strong bones. Walking at a brisk or fast pace benefits bone mass in the hip, walking slowly is not as helpful, the intensity is important. Low-intensity activity might be beneficial for overall strength and fitness but will have less total effect of bone mineral density.

In our busy lives it is difficult to dedicate time to exercise. However, if we can capture the increase in productivity achieved by the decrease in health problems, improved sleep, stamina, mood and mental capacity, the time spent exercising will compensate tremendously. It is important to schedule your time to exercise in your daily routine. If you are a busy working person, you may want to actually schedule it in your day book or planner, and do not let anything interfere with that time. You may also want to plan on meeting a friend at a set time several times a week. If you're a stay-at-home Mom, you especially need to find the time in your busy schedule for yourself. The bottom line is there are no excuses for not exercising. Consider this your sacred time. It is the time when you will connect with yourself, with your body, with your being.

We often struggle to get going in the morning and just the idea of starting to exercise is unbearable when we are under the warm covers, especially in the winter months. It may be helpful to just accept that it is difficult and instead of imagining engaging in the vigorous activity, just imagine being able to slither out of bed and crawl to an area of your room or home where you can do neck and waist rolls, trunk and back stretches and perhaps some marching or leg rises. After a few minutes you have activated your system enough that you will struggle less in pushing yourself out of the house or into the exercise room. It is always an issue of will.

Imagery of past pleasurable physical activities and the knowledge about the benefits of exercise will create the motivation; but it is only the part of you that commands your body to overcome the inertia, your will that will make you change your pattern and create the habit of exercising regularly. It can take repeating a positive action as few as a dozen times to create a new habit; but it will take about three to six months to truly effect change.

Explore and resolve the various concepts and mental constructs that may get in the way of creating the exercise habit. If you have difficulty creating this on your own you may want to consult a counselor or a personal coach to help identify the resistances and overcome the limitations to get your program going effectively.

In order to break the inertia it is very important to visualize times in the past when you have been active and feeling the sense of freedom and power from being engaged in a vigorous activity, such as walking, hiking or jogging. Often, images of playing as a child, or playing sports in school and college can increase motivation to start being more active physically.

As a runner who has been running most of my adult life, I look at my running as 'play'. It's my time to be child-like. If you think of exercise as work, you're not going to want to do it, but if you look to your inner child and make whatever you choose to do a fun experience, you'll be successful, which brings to mind one of my favorite running stories.

For ten years I worked as the Vice President of Marketing for a major financial institution. One of my fondest memories of that job was sneaking out of my office at lunch time in my running shorts, down the back steps, and out a side alley door. It was like playing hooky from work, even though it was my lunch hour. I would put a small stick in the door to hold the lock open so I could get back in unnoticed when I returned forty minutes later, (just enough time to run five miles). This would allow me time to clean up in the men's room and grab a quick lunch at my desk before getting back to work.

One day upon returning, I noticed my stick was missing and the alley door was locked. You can only imagine my initial shock at the time. All I was wearing was a pair of running shorts and shoes, no shirt. My office was on the fifth floor of the building right next to the men's room and the stairway down to the alley door, my secret getaway. In order to get to my office, on that memorable day, I would have to walk through the main lobby of the bank, past the corporate offices, to the elevator, barely dressed, at the busiest time of day. I stood in the alley for what seemed an eternity, gathering up the will to walk through the main lobby. Beginning the very next day, I no longer snuck out the back door. I took the steps and walked proudly past the corporate offices and through the lobby. So find time every day to 'play'; you (and your bones) will be the better for it.

A note on weight training: something else I, (like many) resisted for far too many years, is also in order. As mentioned previously in more than thirty years of running, I experienced every imaginable running injury. In 2004, Christina, a weight training/gym fanatic, purchased three weight training sessions with a personal trainer as a Christmas gift for me. That gift certificate sat on my desk, unused for nearly a year. In December 2005, two weeks prior to Christmas, Christina asked me if I was going to use the gift certificate. If not, she was going to; it was about to expire.

Reluctantly, I arrived at the gym for my first one hour session with Christina's trainer, Al. Alberico Richezza, (what a name, huh?) was pretty big, and equally strong. As you would expect in a South Philly gym (think Rocky), there were a lot of big, strapping guys . . . and women for that matter, to make certain I felt like a fish out of water. All I could think was: "This is why I don't go to the gym." It was all about my own insecurities.

Well, that one training session became three; three became twelve; twelve became twenty-four. Today, while I certainly don't have an 'Arnold' physique, (yet), I am considered one of the 'guys' at the gym. I weight train four days weekly, and have developed muscle and gotten stronger in ways I cannot begin to explain. I stand straighter than I ever have; I run stronger than I have in years, and I feel so much stronger as a result.

To get yourself motivated go out and pick up a copy of the book 'Body for Life' by Bill Phillips. It will inspire and change your life in ways that you can't begin to imagine.

COMPLEMENTARY/ALTERNATIVE APPROACHES

Homeopathic Medicine

Homeopathy is a medical treatment used by thousands of practitioners around the world for about 200 years. It has been used to treat many conditions acute and chronic, from skin rashes and earaches to infections and cancer. Most reports on the efficacy of homeopathy are anecdotal and very few studies have followed current scientific standards. However, many scientists conclude that homeopathy may be of value in the treatment and prevention of diseases in humans, animals and even crops.

Homeopathy is based on the premise that illnesses can be treated with very small dosages of substances capable of producing the same symptoms when taken in large dosages. A homeopath will take the patient's symptoms and compare them with the records of experiments, done by homeopaths, with homeopathic remedies and come up with a remedy that most clearly resembles the symptom picture of the patient.

A homeopath will pay special attention to particular, peculiar and characteristic symptoms, which most other practitioners will dismiss as trivial. Each person will have some distinct manifestation of symptoms even if suffering from a common disorder. Based on those particular differences, a homeopath may choose one remedy or another. Not every person with the flu will need the same remedy. For example, a person with headache that gets better from cold, with thirst for cold drinks but with general chilliness of the body, resembles the remedy picture of the substance phosphorus. A substance like coffee can be used to treat insomnia or onion to treat a cold or hay fever; this is called the "law of similars". Today, researchers are engaged in scientific studies to learn more about how homeopathy works and what conditions are best treated with it.

Homeopaths believe that the symptoms of disease, like inflammation, fever, diarrhea, cough and discharges, are methods the body uses to heal itself and should not be suppressed. These symptoms are used as a guide to understand what is going on with the body and to choose the best remedy to treat the disease at the point in which the organism becomes ineffective in the healing process.

Since these substances can cause the same symptoms as the disease to be treated, homeopaths use very small quantities of remedy to avoid a worsening of the patient. The concentration of the homeopathic remedies is in the range of one part-per-million and at times even more diluted. Sometimes, despite the minuteness of the dosage people may experience an initial aggravation of symptoms that can last a few minutes or up to a few days.

At times, a homeopathic "antidote" is required to reduce the body's reaction and direct it in a more moderate way. Sometimes conventional treatment may be required, especially when the person is suffering or when the condition worsens significantly.

Homeopathic remedies produced according to standards are totally safe and non-toxic. An aggravation is the organism's reaction to the homeopathic stimulus and is not a chemical effect of the medicine but a reaction of the body's susceptibility as it is stimulated by the remedy. It is like going to watch a movie with emotionally charged material. Each person will be affected differently depending on each person's sensitivity and susceptibility.

In a similar manner, the homeopathic remedies will transmit specific information to the body and evoke a reaction from the homeostatic mechanisms of the organism. This explanation is hypothetical and has not been substantiated by concrete research; however there is some basic research probing into the nature of homeopathic dilutions.

Dr. Samuel Hahnemann, the founder of homeopathy, tested his hypothesis of treating people with substances capable of causing the same symptoms by experimenting on himself, his family and a close group of physician friends. He carried out the "proving" (experiment) of ninety-nine substances—mineral, vegetable, and animal—by the time of his death in 1843 at the age of 88.

The symptoms that developed when he or his disciples took the remedies were recorded carefully and classified according to the organic systems these medicinal substances altered, from the mind and general systemic effects, to specific organ systems. In this way, Hahnemann thought, it was possible to determine the specificity and the particular organ affinity of the substances proven. Hahnemann postulated this as a way to discern the actual therapeutic value of medicinal substances, which was lacking in his time.

Today, we have about 2,500 different substances listed in the Homeopathic Pharmacopeia of the United States, the official compendium of homeopathic remedies recognized by the Food, Drug and Cosmetic Act of 1938.

The Homeopathic Healing Process

If your symptoms improve and you are taking a remedy on an on-going basis you need to stop the remedy, wait and observe. The remedies stimulate your own healing systems; once a change occurs, you don't need to stimulate the body any more. If the symptoms return you can re-start the remedy as long as the remedy has been helpful and no other, new, symptoms have appeared. In that way you can start and stop the remedy according to the appearance of symptoms.

At times, several remedies are needed in succession to achieve a complete healing. In acute conditions you may need a different remedy as soon as one hour after the initial remedy. The involvement with homeopathy is more intensive than with conventional therapies.

The symptoms could get worse after the remedy. It is not unusual for the correct remedy to cause a slight and brief aggravation of the symptoms you suffer. Such an aggravation is benign and a good sign. It should be tolerable and last no more than a few hours or up to three or four days. This should be followed by a progressive improvement. Please note that if you are taking a remedy on a regular basis you should stop it if there is an aggravation or as soon as the symptoms start improving noticeably.

If you are taking a remedy regularly and the symptoms become intolerable, if they worsen progressively, or last more than three or four days, stop the remedy and call your doctor. This may mean that the remedy, or the strength of the remedy, is not right for you and some adjustments need to be made.

Sometimes the remedies stimulate your body in a way that brings to the surface certain constitutional vulnerabilities or old, long forgotten, symptoms. This can be a good sign.

I once had a patient who called me two hours after being in my office for a visit during which I gave her the indicated remedy, based on her presenting symptoms. She told me she had suddenly started experiencing a sharp pain in the side of the chest and she was concerned and puzzled by this. I asked her if she had ever experienced a similar pain. She proceeded to tell me that the pain was similar to a time when she was hospitalized acutely for respiratory distress and had a chest tube put through her chest wall. The pain felt just like it had at that time. The pain subsided within several minutes and the patient's initial symptoms improved progressively.

Homeopaths have noticed that in the course of healing the body often goes through old symptoms as if attempting to heal "old wounds" that had not healed completely. These episodes should be mild, tolerable and short-lived and are often called "healing crisis" and are usually a form of a discharge or an eruption. You can continue taking the remedy under these circumstances. As long as the symptoms are not too uncomfortable, it is best to let them run their course. Usually those symptoms don't last more than three or four days. Any significant worsening of symptoms, lasting more than a few minutes or hours; or any persistence of symptoms of more than a few days should be checked in with your doctor.

Finally, in general, you will know the remedy is helping if you notice an improvement in your general well being, your energy, stamina, and emotional state. Local physical symptoms usually are the last ones to improve.

It is said that it takes one month of treatment per year of disease to achieve a cure. Usually it takes about three to six months to assess how homeopathy is working for you. It is recommended to see your homeopath at least three to four times a year when you have noticeable symptoms.

It is best to have a practitioner experienced in homeopathic treatment to take your case and choose the most indicated remedies to your symptoms, not just for osteoporosis, but also all the other organic symptoms including the particular of your organism. Various people suffering from osteoporosis may need a different remedy.

Following, we will describe various remedies described in the homeopathic literature as helpful in the treatment of osteoporosis:

Calcarea Phosphorica: (calcium phosphate)

The person who may need calcarea phosphorica tends to have a generally gloomy, discontent countenance, is fearful and ill-humored. They have intellectual deficiencies with difficulties with memory and intellectual work. They may have arthritic pains that are worse with cold and damp and better from warmth. They tend to be sensitive to drafts of air, with back stiffness and pain. They also suffer with headache caused by being in the cold, which is worse at night and with exertion. They also suffer from sleepiness during the day with sleeplessness at night.

Calcarea Fluorica: (calcium fluoride)

The person in need of this remedy harbors fears of financial instability or inability to get emotional needs met. He/she has a strong need for security and reassurance and tends to be dependant and strongly attached. He/she has anxiety about health with fear of death.

These patients tend to have induration of glands and hard nodular tumors, especially in the breast. They tend to have venous problems and varicose veins. They have nodes in the tendons. The patient tends to have flushes of heat with palpitations. They are aggravated by cold and wet; tends to be better from continuous motion and heat. They are better by eating and aggravated by fasting. They are always hungry and have emaciation with increased appetite.

Often these patients have a history of having had chronic ear infections. Their teeth break and crumble easily; the teeth are loose and have deficient enamel. They are predisposed to hemorrhoids and low back pains. They have rectal fistulas.

They are predisposed to scoliosis and spinal curvatures. They have bone growth called exostoses and have arthritic nodosities. Ligaments are loose and joints tend to be over flexible.

Their perspiration tends to be profuse and offensive and the skin tends to get chapped and cracked.

Silicea

Those in need of this remedy are yielding, mild, refined, and of sensitive temperament. However, they have a desire for self-confidence, tend to be unresolved and timid. They have fears of public speaking, examinations, pointed objects and pins.

This person has a lack of stamina and complains from long mental exertion. They complain of brain fog. They are sensitive, anxious, and even irritable from noise.

They feel worse in the cold, drafts and from being uncovered. They are worse from the suppression of perspiration. They have frequent colds and infections with enlarged glands that may suppurate. They tend to have abscesses and fistulas. They tend to perspire easily from the scalp and neck.

There is a tendency to chronic cough with purulent expectoration and wheezing from cold. They have tendency to pneumonia and are sensitive to cold. They tend to have sensitive nodes of the breast.

They have desires for eggs, fat, ice, ice-cream, cold food and drinks. They tend to have constipation and stool tends to recede, and swelling of the inguinal glands.

They tend to suffer from headaches, especially from the occiput and extending to the forehead. They have the tendency for acute and chronic ear infections, styes in the eyes and purulent discharges. They tend to have impaired hearing, ear stoppage and sinus infections. They tend to have abscess at roots of teeth. Have fistulas and tend to inflammations of the gums. The patients will tend to have Bartholin's cysts and offensive vaginal discharges.

They have tendencies toward scoliosis, spine curvatures, weakness of the back, back pain, sciatic pain and have ailments from injury to the spine. They have a tendency to have brittle nails, rippled with white spots on them. They tend to have ingrown toenails and athletes' feet. They have bunions and swelling around finger nails. They have keloids and scars become painful, stinging and red. There is predisposition to warts.

The dosage of the homeopathic remedies varies depending on the person's sensitivity and susceptibility to disease. In general, it is safe to use the remedies and potencies available in the local pharmacy and health food stores.

Usually homeopathic remedies are available in the natural food stores in various strengths or "potencies". The most common are the 6X, 6C and 30C potency. The 6X dilution can be taken daily, and unless there are any symptoms that arise anew while using the remedies, it can be used for a few months at a time. Of course, it is always ideal to be followed by a practitioner experienced in homeopathic treatment.

CONVENTIONAL THERAPIES

While there are non-pharmacological treatments for osteoporosis, they will not be sufficient to stop or reverse osteoporosis in some people. In these patients conventional medications will be necessary.

Pharmacologic Therapy

Pharmaceutical agents can be classified as antiresorptive agents, that prevent the breakdown of bone, or bone-forming agents, that will add bone mass. Antiresorptive agents include estrogens, selective estrogen-receptor modulators (SERMs), the bisphosphonates, and calcitonin.

Several compounds stimulate bone formation. Parathyroid hormone increases bone density, especially in the lumbar spine. It needs to be administered via subcutaneous injection. Teriparatide (Forteo), a recombinant parathyroid hormone, has been approved for the treatment of osteoporosis in postmenopausal women who are at high risk for fracture and for men with primary or osteoporosis that is a consequence of low gonad function and at high risk for fracture. It is an effective compound, but it has been shown to cause cancer (osteosarcoma) of the bone in experiments with rats, so it is contraindicated in patients with Paget's disease, in people with prior irradiation of the bones, and in those with an elevated alkaline phosphate, an enzyme that marks the degree of bone metabolism and that can be measured in blood. Therefore it is indicated in patients with high risk and only for a short period of time, perhaps no longer than a couple of years.

Fluoride supplementation also stimulates bone formation, but does not decrease risk for fracture, and in fact, higher doses of fluoride seem to increase the fragility of bone. It has not been approved by the FDA for osteoporosis prevention and treatment, and it has been linked to various other physical problems including cancer.

Hormone Therapy

Hormone supplementation therapy (HT) increases bone mineral density (BMD) and prevents bone fractures. However, there has been a decline in the enthusiasm for such therapy because of the potential negative consequences.

Concerns over the benefits of HT were raised after research published in 2002 which showed that it increased cardiovascular disease, stroke, deep venous thrombosis, and breast cancer. The trial was supposed to run for fifteen years, but it was stopped five years early because of the significance of the findings. Combined estrogen/progesterone therapy may provide relief of menopausal symptoms including poor sleep. HT has not shown to improve general well-being, vitality, depression, or sexuality. The long term benefits of the use of HT, or estrogen alone, in women who have had hysterectomy have not been evaluated.

HT will be helpful in women who have had troublesome menopausal symptoms, have had a history of amenorrhea lasting for six months to a year or more, women who have had a premature, surgical or medical menopause, a history of steroid use, a strong family history of osteoporosis, and those who are not responding to alternative treatments, or who can't tolerate other medications. It is important to remark that the bone loss will restart once the estrogens are discontinued at the rate of loss that is usual during menopause.

Progesterone, either synthetic or in the natural form, pill or cream has been shown to increase bone density. There is still some research to be done to confirm the effects of this approach.

Selective Estrogen Receptor Modulators

The FDA approved tamoxifen (Nolvadex) and raloxifene (Evista) in 2000 for the treatment of postmenopausal osteoporosis. These medications have the effect of estrogens in the bone but they are antiestrogenic in the breast tissue. Studies have shown that raloxifene decreases risk for vertebral fracture, but it has not shown to improve fractures outside of the spine.

They also increase the risk of stroke and uterine cancer. These medications cause heat flushes, weight gain, since they block the effects of estrogens. This may pose a problem in women susceptible to dementia. These medications have about the same risk of thrombosis and embolism as estrogens, so these medications are contraindicated in women at risk for deep venous thrombosis. They can also cause leg cramps and skin rash.

Bisphosphonates

Several bisphosphonates have been approved by the FDA for the treatment of postmenopausal osteoporosis, including alendronate (Fosamax), risedronate (Actonel), and in May 2003, ibandronate (Boniva). These medications increase BMD and reduce risk for fractures by interfering with the function of the osteoclasts, the cells in charge of the reabsorption of bone.

These medications are expensive and cause side effects such as nausea, constipation and heartburn. They are associated with inflammation of the esophagus and stomach ulcers in up to one third of patients; however, this may be modulated with the release of once-weekly and once a month regimens, this is yet to be determined. They can also cause headaches, musculoskeletal pain, abdominal pain and diarrhea.

These medications may reduce the risk of fractures by 40% at three to five years. It is important to continue calcium and vitamin D supplements while on these agents. Ibandronate is contraindicated in people who are not able to stand or sit for 60 minutes.

Calcitonin

Derived from salmon, calcitonin is available as a nasal spray and as an injectable preparation. The compound works by regulating the calcium loss in the urine. Side effects include nausea and flushing. Research has shown reduction of the risk of new vertebral fractures with the use of the nasal spray in postmenopausal women with osteoporosis. It has shown to have few side effects but it is not as effective as other medications.

It can produce hypersensitivity and antibody formation, frequent nasal irritation, rhinitis, sinusitis, nose bleeds, back and joint pain, headache, dizziness, flushing, rash, and irritation at the site of injection.

Teriparatide

Teriparatide (recombinant human parathyroid hormone) is the only anabolic osteoporosis medication. Clinical trials show that teriparatide is effective at increasing bone mineral density in the spine and throughout the skeleton by stimulating new bone formation on trabecular, endocortical, and periosteal bone surfaces by stimulating osteoblastic over osteoclastic activity. PTH enhances bone strength by restoring bone architecture in expanding bone size as well as improving bone mineral density.

PTH currently must be administered by subcutaneous injection, although alternative modes of delivery are being investigated. The FDA has approved the use of teriparatide for two years in postmenopausal woman and men at high risk of fracture. It is contraindicated in patients with Paget's disease of the bone or patients with bone metastases or preexisting hypercalcernia. The most common side effects associated with teriparatide include dizziness and leg cramps.

In general, all of these medications may have instances when they are indicated. It is important to discuss the various possibilities with your doctor, and weigh the pros and cons of each treatment approach and medicine. I recommend my patients to follow whatever program is most indicated rigorously, especially if we start with non conventional approaches.

I further recommend my patients to use physical exercise, nutrition and nutritional supplements, and homeopathic, as long as the osteoporosis is not severe. If the patient is an elder, with high risk of fracture, I will recommend a conventional approach. The medicines can then be used until the risk is significantly ameliorated.

I will work with my patients between six months and one year to determine if the non pharmacological approach is sufficient to improve the condition. We will follow progress with DEXA scans and with urinary measures of bone metabolism, the collagen crosslinks, or telopeptides.

Chapter 5

Taking Action

When you are diagnosed with a serious condition, you are forced to deal with a whole new set of rules for your life. In many cases, there is discomfort or outright pain. Your vitality seems to have been drained away in an instant. If facing disability, discomfort and your mortality is not enough to depress you, I am not sure what will. So anyone who minimizes the impact of disease on your psyche has never been seriously ill. In this chapter, we will look at the importance of your mental and emotional health in the recovery of your physical health as you work to decide a course of action to regain the health of your bones.

DECIDING ON APPROPRIATE PHYSICAL TREATMENT

The most appropriate treatment for you will depend, of course, on your age, the severity of your condition, your resources both economical and emotional, and accessibility to treatment.

The treatment of choice depends on various factors. It depends primarily on the degree of impending risk of fracture. A T-score of—2 in a reasonably young woman carries a lesser risk of fracture than a—2 in an 80-year-old woman because of age itself. If you suffer from osteopenia, you certainly have time to try the non-pharmacological and alternative treatments we present here. If you are over 65 and have a severe osteoporosis you may not have more than a few months to try alternative approaches before taking conventional medications.

The best approach for you also depends on your strength of conviction that you can change your condition and have the motivation to do so. It depends on your resources, both financial and emotional, and how much support you have from your family, friends and health practitioners.

At this time, insurance companies do not pay for alternative or complementary treatments; therefore, most of those expenses will be out of pocket. Most of the vitamins and supplements are not covered by insurance, but they are usually not overly expensive. Regardless of the severity of your condition, it will be necessary to add some supplements to your regimen.

As it is important to deal with emotional factors that may affect you, it will be helpful to use psychotherapy to deal with the emotional components of your condition. Most insurance plans will cover psychotherapy to a greater or lesser extent.

If you are suffering from significant emotional distress, like depression or anxiety that is interfering with your life, you may need to add a biological approach. You can try homeopathic medicines and herbs, but you may need conventional medications.

If you are at serious risk of fracture, because of the severity of your condition, or if there is no significant improvement after a reasonable period of time, then conventional medication may be the only resource.

CREATING A PLAN THAT IS RIGHT FOR YOU

Once you, and your doctor, determine your condition and its severity, and you have lined up your resources of practitioners (physician, nutritionist, physical therapist, trainer), and friends who will go out walking and jogging with you, you are ready.

If you have gotten this far in the book you are probably not in denial of your condition and are looking forward to actively work on your program of treatment or prevention. Otherwise, you are reading this book for a dear one who is having a hard time coming to grips with their condition and don't seem to be too motivated to engage in a wholehearted treatment. In that case you may need some extra help. It is hard to deal with denial, when people don't want to take responsibility for their health.

Some of you may decide that all that exercise, physical therapy, training and taking eight or more capsules and tablets of supplements per day is too much; you don't want to bother, and will settle for a bit of walking, some calcium with vitamin D and a conventional medication. Our goal is to give you options.

Identify which are the various components we have presented that appear to suit you and make a list; start with the most critical ones, diet, exercise, calcium, magnesium, vitamin D and reduction of stress. Depending on the severity of your condition and the presence of other complicating conditions, like high cholesterol, homocysteine, arteriosclerosis or arthritis you will need to add red yeast rice, folic acid, B6, vitamin K, MSM, SAMe and/or glucosamine/chondroitin.

If you are feeling overwhelmed at this point, do not despair. It is normal to have these feelings depending on where you are emotionally with your diagnosis and how you deal with issues in your life.

Researchers have looked closely at the process of change in thousands of people engaged in working through a particular behavior that interferes with their ability to be healthy. Whether it is smoking, drinking, eating or procrastination, everybody will approach change from a particular stage and will use similar techniques to move forward toward improvement and/or recovery.

Each of us have a perception about our ability to perform a particular task and will use this measure to determine our ability to perform future tasks. A change in our belief of self-efficacy can predict a lasting change in behavior if there are adequate incentives and skills. We need to believe we can make the change and improve.

If we lack the skill to make the change, like reaching out for help from our practitioners and family with assertiveness, we need to find someone who will help us develop that assertiveness. If we lack the will to get out of bed each morning to exercise we have to get a family member, a friend or a trainer to get us out and exercise. The will is like a muscle, it takes exercise to make it stronger. Initially it takes effort to make changes and assistance can help us in the beginning to get us going and develop some consistency.

Behavior change is often construed as an event, such as quitting smoking, drinking, procrastinating or over-eating, or developing positive habits like exercise. But, change occurs over time. The various schools of therapy are used as a "one-size-fits-all". The truth is that the various styles of psychotherapy have a particular function and application depending on the stage of change in which we find ourselves.

Psychoanalytic therapy is good for increasing insight and consciousness, and arousing emotions; humanistic and existential therapies are good at providing helpful relationships and provide liberation of dysfunctional social constructs and encourages advocacy organizations; gestalt/experiential provide techniques for self evaluation and emotional arousal; cognitive techniques help with self evaluation, and identification and countering of dysfunctional thoughts; behavioral techniques help with planning and developing environmental controls, directing and managing impulses and desires, and setting up of aversive and rewarding components of the program. Depending on what stage of change you are in you may benefit primarily by one technique over another. You may need to find a therapist trained in the particular technique you need or you can find a practitioner who is eclectic and experienced in the various techniques.

In my practice, I will meet with my patient long enough to gather all of the relevant information to understand the primordial issues that need to be addressed, from a physical, emotional and spiritual perspective, and determine what will be the best approach to treatment in collaboration with the patient. Depending on where the patient is emotionally, I may recommend different approaches. Someone who is very insightful and motivated will be able to address more dimensions and follow a more involved treatment program than someone who is not significantly motivated for change, even if in pain, or someone who cannot get activated because of being depressed.

Researchers have found that change is a process that progresses through a series of five stages. These stages are: pre-contemplation, contemplation, preparation, action, maintenance and termination. These stages of change are not always archived in a straight line but more often in a spiral-like trajectory.

In the pre-contemplation stage people usually are not aware or do not want to acknowledge there is a problem. Usually it is the family, friends or coworkers that see the problem. People in this stage usually resist change and use defense mechanisms like denial, blaming others for their problems, or rationalize their behavior to justify their condition and not have to change.

People in this stage are often uninformed or under-informed about their problem or the consequences of their behavior. They may have tried to change several times and become demoralized with their perceived inability to maintain their actions or to change. They tend to avoid reading, talking or thinking about their problem behaviors.

People in this stage are often characterized as resistant or unmotivated or as not ready for health promotion programs. It is only by repeatedly and patiently providing education about the negative consequences or their predicament, proving their rationalizations as erroneous, or when circumstances in their environment force them to change that they will eventually move onto the next stage, that of contemplation.

In the contemplation stage people are able to see that they have a problem, they start to understand it, wonder about possible solutions, but are not ready to make a commitment. It is marked by ambivalence in which the pros and cons of the change are contemplated back and forth. By exploring the rationalizations and excuses for not taking action, the contemplation stage works on removing the emotional and intellectual obstacles to change. Here we need to focus on the solution rather than the problem and on the future rather than the past and being stuck. The end of this stage and the move into the preparation stage is marked by anticipation, excitement, activity and at times anxiety.

In the preparation stage people make the final adjustments before beginning to change their behavior. An important step here is to make our decision to change public. Telling the important people in our lives makes our commitment more serious. There is still ambivalence in this stage and it is important to continue focusing on why the change is important, what will be the outcome, and visualize advancing towards that goal with resolution. Research your condition to get educated about the various options and plans, imagine and feel what it would be like to do one or another activity. This helps to motivate and set the stage for change.

Often we may set the terrain by instituting a number of small behavioral changes, such as we mentioned above, start with the skeleton of what will be the most basic program to deal with your osteoporosis or with your commitment to preventing it from occurring.

It is best not to cut this stage short by impulsively implementing action. It is best to take some time to plan carefully; developing detailed steps and actions, and making sure you know the processes of change that will help you through the maintenance and termination phases.

The people you surround yourself with, the lifestyle activities you engage in, will make your progress easier or harder. If you are used to walking in, or driving by, your local coffee or donut shop to load up on coffee and pastries in the morning, it will take some effort to change your habits. You will need to come up with a different routine and substitute the problem behaviors with others that will move you in the path of recovery and healing.

In the action stage you will see yourself implementing, wholeheartedly, the behaviors you need to have to accomplish your goal. You will have removed the obstacles to your cure, the controllable factors, and implement the ones that will lead to your improvement in health. This is the most active stage; the one that requires the greatest commitment of time and energy. These actions are very visible and you may see the greatest return for your investment.

Nevertheless, it is important to be cautious in this stage. It is risky to interpret an initial bout of action as permanent change and we loose commitment to see that change to the end. Often, the people around us stop giving us encouragement, since they believe we are now successfully changed, and we may lower our guard. Here is where you need to make sure you maintain a high level of awareness of your stage, keep track of your emotions, your self image, your thinking, especially if you identify doubts or negative patterns.

As mentioned above, the stages of change are not linear. Often we may, seemingly, regress to a contemplation or pre-contemplation stage, where we stop the activities that were leading to the resolution of the problem. Do not get discouraged. It is common to regress. The critical thing is to identify that you have slipped and need to get back on track as promptly as possible.

In the maintenance stage the challenge is to maintain the gains you have attained through the hard work of the other stages and work on preventing the lapses and relapses. It is important to find things in your program that are fun and distracting. You need to find things that are emotionally rewarding in order to keep your level of interest and excitement high. Create variety and innovation; modify your routine ever so slightly to prevent getting bored with the program. For example, you can change the order of exercises you perform, run or walk a different route, listen to different music, books on tape or educational programs while you exercise. If any element of your program becomes boring, or if you drop it, you need to meditate on the obstacles or resistances that have appeared in order to solve it.

The termination stage is the ultimate goal for all changes. The former problems are no longer present and are no longer a threat. Here you probably will experience the confidence that you will not relapse into the patterns of your old behaviors. The new behaviors and habits you have created in your life will be continuous and without further significant effort on your part, they become "second nature".

You need to keep track of your progress along the way and determine what stage you are in. In managing osteoporosis you will require periodical laboratory tests to measure the various parameters we mentioned above to ascertain progress. This will help to figure out if the plan should continue or needs to be modified along the way.

If you continue to lose BMD there are considerations you need to keep in mind. The first one, of course, is that you are probably not adhering faithfully to the treatment. But if you are following the program consistently, there is probably poor absorption of the supplements, drugs or there is improper dosing. We always forget about the secondary causes of osteoporosis. True non-responsive patients do exist, and if that were the case, you should consider changing therapies.

Hopefully, you will be able to develop the resources, strength, courage and persistence to move through the various stages of change and treatment towards your total recovery. Just remember, be patient and compassionate with yourself. Loving others and yourself will provide you with strength and incentive to heal.

Part Three

The Diet Connection

Chapter 6

Diet for Healthy Bones

The Yellow Emperor's Classic of Internal Medicine, the foundation of the wisdom of Chinese medicine says this: 'Overindulgence in sweets will cause pain in the bones . . .' In this simple phrase lies the crux of the problem of food and our bone health. If we don't know what causes bone loss; if we don't understand the impact of food choices on our bone health, how can we ever expect to know what to do to prevent or reverse the problem?

While osteoporosis is said to have many 'causes' from menopause to genetics, the most important factor in bone health is how we treat our bodies, most especially what we choose to eat.

What we eat both fuels and drains our body. The notion that our bones just stand there, keeping our bits from collapsing into a heap, is silly at best. The fact is that they are living tissue and the food we choose impacts them both directly and indirectly. The most direct impact is the result of not consuming enough vitamin D, calcium and protein, inhibiting our bones' ability to rebuild themselves. The indirect impact comes because many of our nutrients are inter-related, so a deficiency in one nutrient causes a deficiency in another. And then there are aspects of our diet that impact our bones because they cause an active drain of nutrients, causing deficiencies over time.

ACID AND ALKALINE . . . AN INTERESTING IDEA

You may have heard of the concept of creating a balance of acid and alkaline in the body to create health. It is the basis of many natural healing modalities and is a wonderful concept to understand as you become proactive in maintaining your health.

Acids are simply substance that contain hydrogen atoms that are missing electrons, so they take the needed electrons from somewhere else. That tendency to borrow makes them corrosive by nature. In our body, acids generally result from metabolic processes like breathing and moving, so they are excreted or neutralized by minerals or salts, which are considered to be alkaline.

For proper function of our metabolism, our blood plasma should be slightly alkaline, 7.45 to be exact. This delicate balance is essential to our very existence. Check this out . . . lockjaw or tetanus can cause an alkaline blood plasma pH of 7.9, resulting in death, while a diabetic coma accompanied by a pH of 6.9 will result in death. With the balance, balanced, so to speak, the body is in a state of 'homeostasis,' an inner equilibrium.

It's not just food that keep this balance in check. Our clever body has mechanisms in place that will naturally keep us perfectly balanced. However, our food choices can either support or muck up this process. Our natural check and balance system involves these processes: breathing (which lowers the body's acid load), moving (muscle movement breaks down glycogen to produce energy, increasing the acid load), kidney function (regulates the acid-alkaline balance by excreting a more acid or alkaline urine) . . . our food (you had to know we'd get here) . . . foods contribute to an acidic or alkaline environment once they are metabolized.

Simply stated, protein, carbohydrates, sugar, flour, beans, grains, fish, poultry, meat, eggs and dairy are acid-producing foods. Vegetables, fruits and sea vegetables are alkalizing in the body because they leave behind a residue of minerals in the body.

So what's the key? To maintain health and vitality of our body and bones is dependent upon choosing healthy food options from both the acid and alkaline groups of foods . . . making, you got it . . . balance. Too high a proportion of acid-producing foods will rob our bones of minerals, while too many alkalizing foods will cause us to crave sweet foods and ultimately cause an acid overload. Choosing wisely from each group creates the delicate balance of acid and alkaline that we need for health.

Acid/Alkaline Foods

Acid-forming Foods	Neutral Foods	Alkalizing Foods
Alcohol	Tofu	Juice
Sugar		Fruits
Oils		Green Vegetables
Nuts		Green Beans
Flour		Potatoes
Whole Grains		Root Vegetables
Beans		Sea Plants
Fish		Soy Sauce
Poultry		Miso
Meat		Salt
Eggs		
Dairy		

Even a slight tilt toward acidity in the blood can damage our bones. Called acidosis, this is the perfect environment to remove calcium from the bones to neutralize the acid being produced. Studies have shown that calcium leaves the bones when the environment is too acidic. A study conducted by Dr. T. Colin Campbell in Beijing showed that, in middle aged and elderly women, the consumption of acid-forming foods, like meat, increased calcium excretion in the urine, indicating bone loss. Interestingly, the intake of plant protein showed no such tendency, which could be the reason that vegetarians show less bone loss overall, but if they consume more and more sugar and flour, both acid-producing foods, we may see a different result.

BONE-BOOSTING FOODS

You may be wondering, at this point, however, the true impact of food choices on the health of our bones (and the rest of our bodies). The simple truth is that food is the foundation upon which we build the rest of our health. To minimize the importance of food would be akin to saying that it matters little what type of gasoline we choose to fuel our cars and keep them running at their most efficient.

We are bombarded with marketing for just about everything we consume. We are overwhelmed with evening news sound bites about various studies voicing laundry lists of statistics about what we eat. We are so hammered with information and advertisements that we don't know what to think anymore.

The simple truth is that whole, unprocessed, seasonal, organic (where possible) foods will provide you with the most bang for your nutritional buck, helping you to maintain your day to day health, including your bones. There now, wasn't that easy? No marketing, no ads . . . just my experience.

Okay, so now you are ready to become a proactive partner in regaining the health of your bones. Before you run out the door to go food shopping, keep in mind that there are vegetables that will serve your bones more than others. Here are the best bone boosters I have found.

You will need five to ten servings each and every day of organically grown vegetables (and no, garnish doesn't count as a serving). With so much to choose from, you should have no trouble getting all the yummy vegetables you need, choosing from the following.

Dark Leafy Green Vegetables

Dark leafy greens, cooked and raw . . . kale, collards, mustard greens, broccoli rabe, arugula, watercress, turnip tops, escarole, chicory, bok choy, broccoli, endive, parsley, scallions, etc. Check this out . . . bok choy alone contains 790 milligrams of calcium per 100 calories, 495 milligrams of calcium per 100 calories of cooked mustard greens, compared to 351 milligrams of calcium per

100 calories of skim milk. Getting the picture? Any dark leafy green vegetable you choose will be a rich source of calcium as well as vitamin C, folic acid, magnesium and vitamin D . . . all combined and balanced by Mother Nature herself for our bones.

Roots, Round and Cruciferous Vegetables

Root, round and cruciferous vegetables . . . carrots, parsnips, daikon, sweet potatoes, turnips, rutabaga, winter squash, onions, cabbage, Brussels sprouts, cauliflower, etc. These vegetables are not only delicately sweet, providing us deep satisfaction, but also are rich sources of trace minerals, anti-oxidants, potassium, pantothenic acid and complex carbohydrates.

Other Vegetables

Other vegetables . . . celery, mushrooms, ginger, radishes, chives, leeks, Belgian endive, garlic, avocados (okay, they are a fruit), etc. These vegetables round out our nutritional needs supplying us with everything from essential fatty acids to sodium and antibacterial compounds.

Sea Vegetables

Sea vegetables . . . wakame, hiziki, arame, dulse, nori . . . we could do a lot worse for our health than to follow the example of the Japanese and include mineral-rich sea vegetables in our diet. Rich in magnesium, phosphorus, iron, zinc, calcium and other trace minerals, these powerful foods are only needed in tiny amounts, 5% of your diet . . . to be exact.

And that's just the veggies . . .

Beans

Beans . . . lentils, chickpeas, black beans, split peas, cannellini beans, lima beans, kidney beans, mung beans, etc . . . for rich vegetable sources of protein, complex carbohydrates and fat, as well as calcium, vitamin D, niacin, iron and pantothenic acid.

Nuts and Seeds

Nuts and seeds . . . almonds, walnuts, pecans, hazelnuts, cashews, pumpkin seeds, sunflower seeds, sesame seeds and hempseeds . . . all great sources of protein, trace minerals and fat, including essential fatty acids.

Soy Products

Tofu, tempeh and soymilk are just a few of the wonders of the soyfood family that provide us with phytonutrients (including phytoestrogens), anti-oxidants, protein and fat.

Whole Grains

And then? The best source of fiber, balanced complex carbohydrates, protein and B-vitamins come to us in the form of whole grains, from brown rice and barley to millet, quinoa, buckwheat, corn, wheat, oats, amaranth, etc. Cracked grains are also a great source of fiber and other nutrients . . . corn grits, oatmeal, bulgur, whole wheat bread and pasta.

Fruit

What about fruit? Well, the purist in me wants to say that fruit, eaten in excess, can cause an acidic atmosphere in your blood and inhibit the recovery of your bones' health. I do, however, live in the real world and I know that people love fruit and have a hard time accepting that it might not serve their health. Remember that, while high in fiber, vitamins C, D and K, iron, magnesium, potassium, as well as antioxidants, fruit is also rich in simple sugar, thereby creating an acidic blood condition. Seasonal fruit is best . . . apples and pears in autumn, peaches, berries, melon and apricots in the summer. As for dried fruit, always cook it so that the sugars are gentled and will make less drama in your blood chemistry, sending your glucose levels into the stratosphere, only to crash and burn soon after.

Healthy Fat

Fat? Poor fat . . . over the last several years, fat has taken such a whipping. Good news, bad news, confusing news . . . do we eat it? Avoid it? Is it evil? Good for us?

Fats are one of the three essential macronutrients that provide us with the calories we need. A concentrated form of energy, fat works as the vehicle that transports fat-soluble nutrients, like vitamins A, D, E and K in the body. Good quality fats, in proper balance with the rest of your diet, are essential for the proper function of our immune and hormone systems, cell wall construction, sex hormones and essential fatty acids, omega-3 and omega-6 are closely involved with the metabolism of calcium. And if that's not enough for you, fat is the vehicle responsible for the great, sensual taste of most of our foods.

There are three basic types of fatty acids: "saturated fat," "monounsaturated fat," and "polyunsaturated fat." "Saturated fat," found in animal food, margarine and hydrogenated oils, contains carbon bonds that are covered with hydrogen atoms. These are the fat molecules that our body prefers to use, so these are the fat molecules we store first. When we consume saturated fat, it's stored in our tissue and on the outside of most organs (like our heart and lungs) and as plaque in our arteries. In America, saturated fat is the main contributor to obesity, heart attack, stroke, and many other diseases and conditions. Another fatty acid, *trans*-fatty acid, is chemically similar to saturated fat, but is made by "hydrogenating" or heating a polyunsaturated fat. Although similar, *trans*-fatty acids are far more harmful to the health than even the butter or cheese they replace in our bid for a healthier diet.

"Monounsaturated fat," like that found in avocado, olive, canola, almond, and peanut oils, have a molecular structure which affects allows them to remain more fluid or slippery than saturated fat. This lets them be burned for energy more easily, instead of ending up on our hips and tummies as stored fat. This is a better oil to use for cooking, since monounsaturated fat can't be converted to a *trans*-fatty acid by heating or cooking, unlike polyunsaturated fat.

While most foods have a blend of these three fatty acids, only one is critically needed to sustain life. "Polyunsaturated fat" is found in flax, sunflower, sesame, safflower, soy, walnut, corn, soy and hempseed oils. This is where *omega*-3, *omega*-6, and *omega*-9 (actually a category of non-essential fatty acids, including oleic acid, which makes up 75-80% of olive oil) are found, those "essential fatty acids" required by the body.

What are essential fatty acids? Sometimes called "the good fats," these are the two polyunsaturated fatty acids that must come from our diet, as our body cannot manufacture them. They are *omega*-3 (alpha-linolenic acid) and *omega*-6 (linoleic acid). (A derivative of linoleic acid (*omega*-6), is gamma-linolenic acid or GLA. Good sources of GLA include hempseed and hempseed oil, blue green algae, spirulina, evening primrose oil, black currant seed oil, borage oil and some fungal oils. Research has shown it to alleviate symptoms of psoriasis, atopic eczema and mastalgia. It has also been under investigation for its beneficial effects on cardiovascular, psychiatric and immunological disorders.)

Essential fatty acids are the raw materials for the cells and are needed for all of the body's functions. Essential fatty acids are vital to the long-term maintenance of healthy human tissue, promoting the healthy function of our brain, heart, digestive and immune systems. The ideal balance of these essential fats is one key to our health. The recommended ratio, three parts *omega*-6 to one part *omega*-3 is not as easy to obtain as it sounds.

Omega-6 is very common, found in most foods from meat and dairy products, to nuts and seeds. We really have no problem getting enough *omega*-6 in our diet, unless of course, we are eating a low-fat diet. *Omega*-6 is needed for blood clotting, proper circulation, healthy kidney and liver function, and proper healing of internal injury. A deficiency in *omega*-6 can result in increased blood pressure and cholesterol levels, hardening of the arteries and artery obstruction, arthritis, poor circulation, premenstrual syndrome, reduced sperm production, slow growth and wound healing and a variety of skin disorders. However, since it's abundantly found in most people's diets, there isn't much worry about getting it. Most American diets have too much *omega*-6 and too little *omega*-3, throwing off the delicate balance necessary to health.

Omega-3 is a fatty acid not as easy to get. Found only in fish and some vegetables, nuts and seeds, the effects of *omega*-3 deficiencies are becoming an epidemic in our modern world. Although we need only small amounts of this powerful essential fat, it is responsible for all vital body functions, including the fluidity of our blood, increased immune function, balance of cholesterol production, proper growth, fetal development, mental acuity and cell renewal. A deficiency of *omega*-3 can cause such problems as arrhythmia, asthma, arteriosclerosis, attention deficit disorder, bipolar disorder, bone loss, breast cancer, colon cancer, diabetes, hypertension, inflammation, immune disorder, migraine headaches, obesity, prostate cancer and psoriasis . . . to name but a few!

Fat-free and low-fat diets further reduce the amount of *omega*-3, making us feel hungry and deprived. We might binge on high-calorie foods to compensate for the deficiency of fat and *omega*-3, and eating less fat inhibits the absorption of fat-soluble nutrients (including vitamins A,D, E and K). But a diet high in *omega*-3 can result in softer skin and stronger hair, natural weight loss, improved memory, improved vision, faster wound healing, more energy, improved vitality, and more.

Just about everyone is aware that a diet high in saturated fats, like those found in meat, dairy foods and hydrogenated oils, causes plaque in the arteries, reduces blood flow, and increases the risk of heart attack and stroke. But not all polyunsaturated fat is created equal. If it's been hydrogenated or partially hydrogenated, the oil has become a *trans*-fat and will not have the benefits to our health of the essential fatty acids, plus it is seen by our body as a saturated fat. All in all, a waste of a good polyunsaturated fat, I'd say.

Essential fatty acids make blood platelets less sticky, so they don't cause hardening of the arteries, like *trans*-fat and saturated fat. Essential fatty acids are too important to the body to be used for mere energy storage, like the other fats. It would seem that there's only good news here! The building blocks for all of the body's biochemicals, including hormones and prostaglandins, are essential fatty acids. They also help carry toxins from the skin, kidneys, lungs and intestinal tract, and create energy within the cells by delivering oxygen from red blood cells.

Essential fatty acids are made into the hormone, prostaglandin, which controls cholesterol production and blood platelet aggregation. As the different prostaglandins made from the different essential fatty acids often have opposite effects in the body, their delicate balance is best obtained from a source closest to the 3:1 *omega*-6-to-*omega*-3 ratio.

So how do we get these essential fatty acids in our diet? As I said earlier, *omega*-6 isn't much of a problem to get, but *omega*-3 is. Additionally, it's important that we eat the proper balance of these two fats. With no essential fatty acids present in meat or dairy products, coldwater fish, and especially salmon, are rich in both essential fatty acids, but in particular the illusive *omega*-3. But as the controversy around fish continues to grow, it needs to be re-thought. Our oceans and rivers grow more polluted, and the toxins from the water can be found in the fatty flesh of the fish. Fish is increasingly farm-raised, with diminished levels of the *omega*-3 we desperately need.

As a vegetarian or vegan, sources of *omega*-3 are even more scarce. With trace amounts in avocados, walnuts and pumpkin seeds, many have looked to flax oil, flax seed and other supplements. However, that's changing. For the last several years, there has been a slow resurgence of an ancient food, hempseed, which supplies as much as 20% *omega*-3, and in the optimal 3:1 ratio for best health. High in complete protein and amino acids, this super plant food has become my primary source of obtaining essential fatty acids in my diet. Delicious, easy to use and completely versatile (which you'll see in a variety of the recipes in this book), hempseed and hempseed oil can help us to obtain the fats essential to our good health and vitality.

All this being said, there's good news and bad news about fat. A diet extremely high in fat, saturated and otherwise, can contribute to osteoporosis, while a diet extremely low in fat can also contribute to osteoporosis. A combination of good quality fats, used moderately, will ensure strong bones and overall good health.

BONE 'WASTERS'

We understand that a lack of certain nutrients will result in bone loss, since we have less building material. But it's as important to understand that using up what nutrients we take in . . . and more . . . will do the same. Here are just some of the ways in which we deplete our bones of the nutrients they need to stay strong and dense.

Simple Carbohydrates . . . and Sugar

Acid-forming foods create a tendency toward acidosis in the bloodstream and to counteract this, calcium and other minerals will be withdrawn from the bones. Bone reduction increases to rebalance the blood and calcium and other minerals are excreted in the urine. Of course, an increase in alkalizing foods will help to neutralize the equation by replacing lost minerals that have been leached from the bones. However, most modern diets are sorely lacking in vegetables and other mineral-rich foods and if these circumstances persist year after year, the amount of calcium and other minerals lost will result in severe bone loss.

Let me be perfectly clear on this point. Carbohydrates are seriously acid-producing foods, considering that their metabolic byproducts include carbonic acid. However, before you rejoice in not eating carbohydrates, let me continue. Whole grains, like brown rice, barley and whole wheat have fiber, trace minerals and vitamin E in them, which reduce the acidifying effects. Simple, refined carbohydrates have none of these saving graces and simply rob us of the nutrients we need for healthy bones. Their acidifying effects are, in fact, enhanced by their lack of minerals. So the regular consumption of white flour, white rice and white sugar will contribute in a major way to bone thinning and weakness.

Of all these simple carbs, though, white sugar is the worst offender and the worst for our bone health. This devitalized food, according to Robert Crayhon, author of 'Nutrition Made Simple' is the cause of a litany of what ails us . . . including bone loss. Look at this list! Refined white sugar is responsible for:

Raising the insulin level and contributing to diabetes
Raising blood pressure, cholesterol and triglycerides, contributing to
    cardiovascular disease
Contributing to the formation of gallstones
Contributing to obesity
Contributing to mood swings and depression
Creating increased stomach acid
Contributing to migraine headaches
Weakening immune function
Depleting our bodies of B vitamins, calcium and copper
Interfering with the absorption of calcium and magnesium

These last two are major contributing factors in the creation of osteoporosis. Yet, despite what we know . . . and we all know sugar is not great for our health, we moan and whine about being 'deprived' when we can't have it as a part of our regular diet.

Simple sugars, from those sparkling little white crystals, to fruit and juices, are simple carbohydrates, composed of loosely bound molecules of glucose, unlike complex carbohydrates, composed of tightly bound chains of glucose molecules. The difference in our bodies is like night and day and the difficulty lies in the amount of simple carbohydrates that we consume versus the amount of complex carbohydrates.

Refined sugar is found, of course, in the obvious places, candies, chocolate bars, soft drinks and other snack foods. I can hear many of you saying, "But I don't eat that stuff". Just read a few labels. Sugar is an ingredient in so many other products, from breads and pasta to cereals to salad dressings and sauces and other processed foods, that we are consuming tremendous amounts of simple, refined sugar without actually eating junk food. From maple syrup, high fructose corn syrup, fructose, sucrose, molasses and other simple sugars, many natural products contain as much simple sugar as any junk food snack.

The molecular structure of simple sugar, causes them to be rapidly absorbed into the bloodstream, causing the glucose level to rise very quickly. When this happens, the pancreas (the organ that regulates blood sugar) secretes insulin that moves excess sugar from the blood to the cells. With this, blood sugar drops, resulting in rapid fluctuations in metabolism what we know as sugar 'highs' and 'lows,' as the levels of glucose in the blood rise and fall erratically. We experience a burst of energy as the levels of glucose rise, followed by the inevitable crash, as the glucose levels drop, leaving us feeling depleted and tired.

If we continue this pattern over time, the body grows exhausted from the extreme levels of energy, as well as the sugar robbing our bones of calcium and other essential minerals and contributing to the loosening of tissue and muscle, leaving us looking weak and puffy, overweight and lethargic. How sweet it isn't . . .

Caffeine

Ahhh, caffeine . . . that substance that gives us such a rush. We savor that first cup of coffee, dependent on it to get moving in the morning, continuing its direct impact on us with sodas, diet sodas and chocolate throughout the day.

Want to know how your morning cup of java, your diet soda with lunch and your daily candy bar could be wasting your bones? Studies show that women with a higher intake of caffeine were at risk of hip fracture at a rate three times higher than those women not taking in caffeine.

Caffeine consumption increases the excretion of calcium and magnesium through the urine, indicating bone loss. The good news is that young women can compensate pretty well for this loss, since they absorb calcium pretty well in the intestines. Older women, however, are at a distinct disadvantage.

So how much caffeine is too much? A lifetime of the equivalent of two cups of coffee a day has been associated with decreased bone density at the spine and hip. Even decaffeinated coffee is highly acidic, so I am not sure you are any better off with that as your choice. And if you pile the sheer volume of soda, diet soda and chocolate we eat on top of two cups of coffee and you have created the perfect environment for osteoporosis.

So are doomed to no coffee or chocolate? Nah, but we do need to be conscious of how much we consume . . . small amounts are most likely harmless. And soda? Even a sip is deadly, but that's me.

Saturated Fat and Cholesterol

In most of the industrialized world, fat accounts for about 40-45 percent of our daily diets. Now I know we need fat for normal body function, but really . . . In the form of hardened, saturated fats, like those found in hamburgers, pizza, fried foods, dairy products, meat, eggs and junk snack foods, these fats (and cholesterol) accumulate in various organs and tissue, clog blood vessels and inhibit body functions. With fat accumulating and hardening in various places within our system, the flow of vitalizing energy is inhibited and blocked and nutrients can not be properly assimilated and minerals are lost in the process of digesting these hard, dense fats.

Protein

What? Protein bad for our bones? I thought we needed it. Hang on . . . after saturated fat and cholesterol, we have to address the intake of protein, so it all makes sense. Sure our bodies and bones need protein to aid in rebuilding. Too little protein, as we know, results in an excessively thin body, with a hollowed out look, a loss of muscle and bone density and overall weakness. However, for most of us, our problems with health come from too much protein, rather than too little.

In adults, our primary requirement of nutrition is to create fuel to carry us through our daily activities, with the secondary job of forming and maintaining cells, which is the primary job of nutrients in children. That means that we require fuel that can be efficiently burned to keep us going. Complex carbohydrates are our best burning fuel. Protein is used in the body to repair, construct and maintain tissue. As adults, most of us require more carbohydrate energy than protein energy for robust health. The problem with carbohydrates comes, as we saw earlier when the quality of the carbohydrates is poor, like white flour.

We require protein for strength and maintenance of our muscles. Without it, we grow weak, with sunken cheeks and an overly thin body. Without sufficient protein, our body will begin to feed on its own muscle for maintenance and strength. But how much is enough . . . and when is it too much? With all we know of nutrition, we are still quite perplexed by protein and how much each person requires. There seems to be no explanation as to why everyone seems to require differing amounts to be healthy. Why do some people require protein at both lunch and dinner to maintain vitality, while others feel lethargic after a protein lunch? I think that protein is quite personal and that we must look at our lifestyle, activity level and needs to decide how much protein we need to maintain our vitality. But back to our bones.

While protein is quite important to our nutrition and maintenance of our vitality, we must understand it. As with everything in nature, there is a front and back to the wonder food . . . protein. Compared to carbohydrates, protein is an inefficient fuel, causing the body to work quite hard to assimilate it and utilize the nutrients in it, which is why high protein diets are so incredibly effective for quick weight loss. The body kicks into high gear and burns tremendous amounts of its resources to break down the density of protein-rich foods. Great, right? Well, for a quick fix for weight loss, you might think so, but the reality of the situation is that protein, in large quantities, can have negative long-term effects on our health.

Animal foods, the most popular source of protein in our modern culture, are highly unstable. Decomposing rapidly, animal foods become toxic, with a virtual plethora of poisons being created in the body as a result. From uric acid to ammonia to sulfates to toxic bacteria, animal protein creates an internal environment akin to a landfill. The kidneys and intestines, our body's key organs for discharge of waste, are overworked and exhausted, growing weak in their ability to do their job. The result? Toxins build up in the bloodstream and in various organs and tissue, leaving us depleted and tired.

The downside of excessive protein consumption can have an even darker side, however . . . the health of our bones. The nutrient in the body that most effectively aids the body in assimilation of protein is calcium. The more dense the protein, the more calcium the body will use in the assimilation process. As more protein is consumed, more calcium is leeched from the bones. The more calcium we lose to this process, the thinner and weaker our bones become, with the risk of osteoporosis a real threat. In a culture where we consume so much protein, we are plagued by calcium deficiencies, supplementing our diet with more and more milligrams of calcium in a futile attempt to stop losing this precious nutrient. Studies have shown that women consuming a diet that leans more towards plant food, rather than animal food (not necessarily vegetarian), show far less occurrences of bone degeneration than their sisters consuming more protein. Ironically, as simplistic as it sounds, if we would simply cut back our intake of dense protein, we wouldn't require calcium supplementing on such an obsessive scale. Our bodies would make a natural balance and our bones would be healthy for our entire lifetime. We would stand tall and strong, with elegant spines and a vital glow.

Dairy Products

Now many experts will classify dairy products, milk, cheese, yogurt and butter as 'buffer' foods for our bones, meaning that they can be used to stabilize the acid and alkaline balance in our bodies. And technically, that may be true if dairy products are used in small amounts. In our culture, excess has, once again, changed that with regard to our health.

Milk is considered to be the perfect food, rich in calcium and protein. Finally, some experts are questioning the wisdom of this thinking. Studies are beginning to show that dairy food is instrumental in causing compromised immune function, allergies, brittle bones, obesity, a variety of reproductive disorders and early onset of puberty.

Mother's milk is our first food, imprinting on us the characteristics and behavior patterns that make us who we are. Does milk contain all the nutrients vital to life? Yes. Species create the perfect milk for their young . . . *their* young. We are the only species that drinks the milk of another after weaning, with the exception of domesticated animals.

The problems associated with drinking milk after infancy reads like a laundry list. Saturated fats and cholesterol in milk clog arteries, contributing to heart disease. The basic milk molecule, casein, is dense, stressing the liver, pancreas, stomach and intestines in the milk drinker. To combat udder infection, commercial dairy cows are fed antibiotics, which in turn attack the flora and villi in the intestines of the consumer, contributing to digestive trouble, just the way second-hand smoke affects the lungs of non-smokers. The estrogen being fed to dairy cows has been directly linked to breast and prostate cancer.

Then there are the children. Commercial dairy cows are pushed to produce more milk than is natural, fed hormones, including estrogen, prolactin and progesterone. In a recent study, it was concluded that the onset of puberty, as early as age ten, is caused by excessive amounts of hormones that children are ingesting in commercial meat and dairy foods. Our children are having children because their bodies are ready too soon.

What about organic milk? Isn't it better? Of course. At the very least, we aren't taking in antibiotics, herbicides, pesticides and hormones, but it's still milk and even without additives, is the root of many problems, including osteoporosis. With the USDA organic standards in place, we can now be sure, as consumers that organic animal products are exactly that, since prior to these standards, none existed for animal food, as they did for fruits and vegetables. Still, milk is not a natural food for mature adults to be consuming. It's for babies, to help them to mature and grow.

What about calcium? Milk is loaded with it, but it doesn't do us much good. The calcium present in dairy is bonded to casein, and although abundant, is largely unavailable to us, since milk lacks magnesium, potassium and vitamin D, unless artificially enriched with these added nutrients.

There's more to it than calcium. Milk protein is dense, designed to build a huge, heavy animal that matures quickly, making it difficult to digest. Animal proteins cause a greater excretion of urea from the kidneys, depleting the body of calcium, magnesium and potassium. The excessive intake of protein causes the blood to become highly acidic. The body relies on serum calcium in the blood to balance that acid, depleting our store of calcium and creating need for supplementation to replenish our loss.

Then there's skim or no-fat milk. By removing the fat, you concentrate the proteins and remove the very component needed for assimilation—fat. The more concentrated the protein, the more calcium is excreted during digestion. By removing the fat, you inhibit the body's ability to assimilate vitamin D, which is vital to our utilization of calcium. Does a body good? Don't be too sure.

The Salt of the Earth

While a necessary ingredient to life, salt has two very different sides to its nature. Literally vital to our existence, natural salt is rich in trace minerals and sodium chloride that are necessary to the health of our blood and essential to our bones, with its alkalizing nature. But that's natural sea salt. But then we have commercial table salt . . . the kind found in snack foods like potato chips, popcorn, salted nuts and processed foods and meats. This salt, far removed from its natural state in the sea, has been stripped of nutrients, re-enriched with its nutrients and laced through with chemicals and preservatives. In this state, even small amounts of salt will have a most dramatic effect on our blood chemistry and bone health, as its alkalizing nature turns highly acidic.

Think about salt with regard to cooking. Sprinkled on food as it cooks, salt causes contraction, sealing in the flavor of each ingredient, while forcing liquid from the food, intensifying the taste. Well, it works similarly in the body. Natural salt, used in appropriate quantities in cooking, helps keep the body strong, with healthy blood, as our muscles and body tissue contract slightly. Used well, natural salt can also help our body hold on to essential nutrients that are key to bone health.

Over time, if excessive use of commercial salt . . . and even natural salt . . . continues, we will see signs of degeneration in our bones, as the salt dries the body, inhibiting the absorption of vitamins and minerals essential to bone health and strength. We will lose our ability to stand tall and straight, as our bones grow brittle and weak.

Moderate use of salt, in cooking, not only adds to the pleasure of eating food, but starts the process of digestion, causing the food to soften as we apply the heat of cooking. Natural, unrefined sea salt, naturally aged soy sauce and miso are the best choices for use of salt. That being said avoid sprinkling salt or soy sauce on cooked food at the table. Raw salt, added to food will only succeed in making our muscles tight and hard, our skin dry and our joints inflexible. However, used delicately in cooking, salt makes eating a pleasure, our blood healthy, our muscles strong and our bones will remain strong.

Nightshade Vegetables

While I am an advocate of the thinking that there is not a vegetable on earth that will kill us, there are some vegetables that we may need to re-think when we are working to reverse a condition as serious as osteoporosis.

The nightshades are a botanical family of plants, called Solanaceae, comprising more than 1700 different plants, some of which are considered to be poisonous, like deadly nightshade . . . or medicinal, like belladonna.

Included among the food plants in this classification include, potato, tomato, eggplant and peppers (red, green, hot, sweet, chili, jalapeno, etc . . . not black or white pepper). Usually associated with arthritis and stiff joints, the nightshades contain 'alkaloids,' compounds that can disturb calcium metabolism. Many studies have shown that minimizing the intake of nightshades results in dramatic abatement of symptoms and discomfort.

Acidic by nature, nightshades have not bee directly linked to osteoporosis, but they have been linked with magnesium imbalance, so it's best to minimize them if you are experiencing bone and joint trouble.

However, if your life will not continue without tomatoes or peppers, here's a little advice. Avoid potatoes completely, as it is nearly impossible to neutralize the acids. If eggplant is your thing, then soak it in salted water for at least an hour to pull the acids from the plant.

Tomatoes and peppers are easier to deal with. The problematic acid resides very close the skin and can be easily neutralized. Take your lead from the Greeks and Italians . . . and what they have traditionally done for generations to rid these foods of 'acida.' Roast peppers over an open flame to remove the outer skin and with it, the acid. With tomatoes, blanche them to remove the skin, use them in sun-dried form or simply marinate them in olive oil, vinegar or lemon juice, salt and black pepper. This simple process draws the acid into the marinade alleviating the problem.

However, if you are struggling with bone loss or thinning and are working to reverse the problem naturally, it may be best to avoid these lovely little plants for a while.

The Junk Food Diet

It used to be that our meals were centered around foods that were seasonal, naturally processed and whole. From animal foods to seasonal vegetables and fruits, our diet was easier on our bodies, with fewer artificial ingredients and additives that made them difficult to digest and utilize. Sadly, our modern culture has replaced fresh, vital foods with processed, refined versions of their natural selves. While these foods may be easy on our lifestyle, they're murder on our health and bones.

Processed foods have been stripped of the light of the sun, the kiss of the breeze and the refreshment of natural water. We eat them and our bodies may receive the vitamins, protein and carbohydrates, but these kinds of foods . . . canned, processed, refined, frozen . . . are devoid of the life energy that sustains us. Processed foods also leave us hungry . . . starving, in fact. When we eat foods devoid of life, we are left dissatisfied with our meals. Not sated, we look for more food. The cycle continues, with us eating more and more quantity. The result is obvious. The more refined foods we eat, the more calories we consume, the heavier we get.

When we eat fresh food, elegantly and simply prepared, the vitality comes through. We are almost overwhelmed by the symphony of flavors that nature provides for our nourishment. Each bite reminds us of the wonder of our world. Our intestines and kidneys eliminate waste efficiently, without excessive loss of minerals essential to bone density and health.

Weight Loss and Low Fat Diets

One of the major risk factors for osteoporosis is being too thin, especially for women and athletes, like distance runners. People can be too thin for varying reasons, food restriction, careless, non-nutritious eating, weight control, health, spiritual or political reasons, as well as reasons beyond the scope of this book.

To understand the impact of weight loss on our bones let's look at weight gain. Most women put on weight after menopause, much to their dismay. However, once the ovaries stop producing estrogen, women's bodies still manufacture a bit from subcutaneous fat, particularly abdominal fat. So in and after menopause, a little extra fat is actually a good thing for our bones because of the continued production of natural estrogen. And ironically, the little bit of extra strain that comes with carrying that weight is actually like a little weight-bearing exercise for our bones.

Now, while I am not in any way promoting obesity, studies out of the National Institute on Aging show that women 50 and over who lose 10% or more of their body fat have twice the risk of hip fracture than women who carry a bit of extra weight. And then there are low fat diets, eating plans restricting the intake of fat so as to reach a certain weight. Weight loss by way of fat restriction fires a direct hit on our bones and is directly linked to loss of bone mass. Here's why. Extremely low-fat diets inhibit the absorption of many fat soluble nutrients, the most important of which, to our bones anyway, is vitamin D. This one nutrient, vitamin D is responsible for the body being able to absorb calcium from the intestines. So a long term restriction of healthy fats in our diets result in bone thinning since the body can obtain and utilize the calcium it needs for bone health due to a deficiency in vitamin D.

A Word About Alcohol

While the occasional glass of red wine or beer can enhance our health and well-being, relax us and provide nutrients, like polyphenols and tannins, for our vitality, excessive intake of alcohol can rob our bones of nutrients and minerals.

In moderation, alcohol will do us no harm, but if it has become a food group for you . . . you know the drill, the nightly martini, followed by a bottle of wine at dinner and then an after-dinner beer, you might want to re-think it. That kind of acid intake will leave you hung over with thin brittle bones.

Keeping Our Bones Strong . . . The Natural Way

We have seen here that there is good news and bad news when it comes to our food choices and our bones. Healing our bodies the natural way requires information, discipline and commitment to ourselves.

In this modern world of ours, all we ever talk about is early detection and relief of symptoms. Cure of any disease is said to come only in the form a small pill . . . brightly colored and marketed by pharmaceutical companies with happy people running in fields of flowers, while the ominous disclaimer is quietly read as a voice-over. Prevention has been relegated to the shadowy world of alternative medicine along with natural cures and remedies. A sad state of affairs for us as humans, I say.

When the world is in a natural state, we can glean all our necessary nutrients from the abundance and variety that nature provides. Traditional societies as far back as we can trace lived well for many generations on abundant nutritious foods. Archeological digs from the fourth century reveal that the people of that time lived at a higher standard of living than we do now . . . at least with food.

Our Food Quality

In our civilized, modern world (and sometimes I use those terms loosely), our food quality is not nearly as high as it could be . . . and not nearly as good as it was a thousand years ago. Over-farming, artificial fertilizers, pesticides, herbicides and fungicides have been some of the largest contributors to the degeneration and demineralization of our soil, resulting in fewer nutrients in the food the land yields.

Much of the food we eat in our modern, can't-be-fast-enough culture are refined and stripped of their naturally occurring nutrients, processed, canned, frozen, artificially colored and flavored, with a large number of chemicals added for . . . whatever reason.

And last, many modern people are in poor health, whether they know it or not, whether they experience acute symptoms or not. A diet of poor quality foods, processed foods, fast foods and other varieties of junk food has compromised our ability to absorb nutrients from food, leaving us weak, tired, with compromised immune function.

What We Do

So what do we do? Are we doomed to a life of swallowing pills? While these three factors have been a great boost to the supplement industry, we can still get most of what we need from our food. And while supplements are, in many cases, necessary and successful, we must never lose sight of the simple fact that our food is our best medicine.

The bad news is that to get what you need from food, you have to be willing to go into the kitchen, get your hands dirty, work up a little sweat and slice and dice, sauté and simmer your way back to health. It's not the easy way, but it is the way that can be sustained, healthfully and deliciously, for a lifetime.

What do we choose so that we know we are getting the most nutrients from our food? When shopping, always look for organically grown and produced foods. This means that they are grown and produced by traditional methods and are free of artificial pesticides, herbicides, fungicides, sewage sludge, growth hormones and antibiotics . . . and have been for at least three years. Recent studies have shown that organically grown vegetables and fruit are 20-30% higher in minerals than commercially grown produce. Farmers' markets, natural foods stores and many supermarkets have a great variety of organically produced foods now, so finding them is not a problem. And the cost? As the demand increases, as consumers demand better quality, organic prices have dropped dramatically, falling in line with the prices of commercially grown produce. No more excuses.

Choose foods that are unprocessed or minimally processed to get the most bang for your nutritionally buck. Natural foods stores, even some supermarkets carry a wide variety of unrefined, whole foods, like whole grains, whole grain breads, whole wheat pasta, beans, fresh vegetables and fruit (not canned, jarred or frozen), nuts, seeds and organically produced animal products, should you choose to eat them.

Most importantly, you have to be willing to go into the kitchen, get your hands dirty, work up a little sweat and slice, dice, sauté and simmer your way back to health. It may not be the easiest way, but it is the way that can be sustained, healthfully and deliciously, for a lifetime.

Cook your food with love and attention and caring. In our modern culture, cooking has been relegated to just another chore at the end of a busy day. For me, cooking is about far more than the process of combining ingredients so that we can eat a meal. Cooking is not just a time-consuming means to an end. Cooking itself is a healing, nourishing meditation.

By cooking, we share in Mother Nature's abundance and her unconditional ability to nourish us. Gorgeous winter squash, its vibrant orange flesh as vivid as the sun that gave it color, hearty carrots as sweet as the earth that cradles them, leafy greens stretching luxuriously open to the rain drops that quench their thirst, whole cereal grains that wave in the gentle breeze that lifts them to maturity . . . our food is a gift from the earth that sustains us. We sell ourselves short if we see cooking food as simply a way to feed ourselves. Handling food is an expression of sincerity and appreciation for the gifts of our lives.

Cooking provides a vehicle for making our lives whole. We have forgotten what truly nourishes us. Our food joins with us, becomes us, helps to create our characters and our health . . . from the bones out. You are alive with vibrant energy . . . recreating yourself and your health, meal to meal.

Can You Do It With Diet Alone?

In a word . . . no . . . not in my opinion, not once you have been diagnosed with severe bone loss. Okay, maybe some people can . . . I am sure there are cases where people have reversed their osteoporosis with diet alone, but those would be rare and unusual cases. And trust me, I know about the power of diet and food choices in our lives and their impact on our health and vitality.

In a perfect world, with perfect food and perfect diligence in the kitchen, you might be able to reverse your osteoporosis with diet alone over a long period of time. Heaven knows, I would never discourage anyone from taking the most natural path to health. But my experience with Robert, in this situation, showed me that a marriage between well prepared healthy food and some supplementation meant his full recovery with no pharmaceuticals.

Based on the severity of your condition, you will need to seriously consider your level of risk before deciding what path to take. In the early stages of osteopenia, you bet . . . diet alone can do the job. Once you have gotten to a severe stage of osteoporosis, you may be a such a high risk of fracture, that you simply do not have time to reverse your condition without supplements. Pharmaceuticals are always the last choice for me, but they may need to be considered, even with your diet change to ensure stronger bones.

The bottom line is simple. We all know our bodies and what is really going on. We may not like it or want to face it, but we know . . . down to our bones, so to speak. Don't let anyone's theory or dogma or personal beliefs alter the path of your own intuition. Listen, gather information, understand your personal condition and how you respond to treatments. Reflect on your health and commit to yourself to be a proactive participant in the regaining of it. Then, you will listen to the only expert on you and your health . . . you.

Chapter 7

Strengthening Soups

The ingredients you put together to make soups can be designed. Don't think of soup in connection to your bones? You should. The starter course to the meal, soup sets the tone for the rest of the meal that will follow, but that's only the beginning of the wonders of soup.

Soup's affect in the body is quite profound, being largely responsible for how well we digest the meal we eat. Try an experiment. Begin dinner with soup one day and without, the next. Really observe the difference in how you assimilated the food you consumed on each day. Were you hungry an hour after dinner or did you remain sated all evening?

Soup works in the body to efficiently draw warming energy into the digestive tract, relaxing and stimulating its function, so that when you eat the solid foods in the main meal, the process of digestion is already at work. Great for digestion, you say, but how does that make for strong bones? When the body can digest food easily, the process of digestion is smoother, more efficient. More efficient digestion means that every cell is receiving the maximum amount of nutrients from our food . . . and that is the basis of vibrant health and strong bones.

Here's how it works. The liquid of the soup does the obvious. Being warm, it relaxes the body, readying it for solid food. When the body relaxes, it can open and release ki or life force, enlivening us with living energy. And by drawing the energy of the ingredients deep into the body, their energy works more profoundly.

The ingredients you put together to make soups can be designed to give your body what it needs most. In need of calcium? How about a light miso soup with a bit of sea plant for minerals, topped off with some sautéed dark leafy greens for a hit of useable calcium? Need some strength and stamina? A hearty soup with some whole grain and sweetly strengthening root vegetables will provide the endurance you need to meet life's little challenges.

By consuming these foods in soup, they have the advantage of the liquid vehicle, so they travel more easily into the body, working effectively and since the body is relaxed, their nutrients and energy can penetrate more deeply to give you the result you want. Understanding the character and energy of the ingredients you choose to make soup will help you to create soups that will take you where you want to go.

So make a fresh pot of soup every day. Savor its deep nourishment and delicious energy—and stay strong.

Pinto Bean Soup with Pine Nut Pesto

A richly flavored bean soup high in protein and loaded with trace minerals essential to building and maintaining healthy bones.

Extra virgin olive oil
3 cloves fresh garlic, thinly sliced
1 small red onion, diced
sea salt
generous pinch crushed red pepper flakes
1-2 stalks celery, diced
1 carrot, diced
1, 16-ounce can diced tomatoes, unsalted
1 cup pinto beans, sorted, rinsed well
1 bay leaf
4 cups spring or filtered water
2 teaspoons white miso

pine nut pesto:
1 bunch fresh parsley, coarsely chopped
1 cup pine nuts
2 cloves fresh garlic, peeled
1/3 cup extra virgin olive oil
1 teaspoon white miso
1 teaspoon brown rice syrup

Place a small amount of oil, the garlic and onion in a medium soup pot over medium heat. When the onion begins to sizzle, add a pinch of salt and red pepper flakes and sauté for 1-2 minutes. Stir in celery and carrot, another pinch of salt and sauté for 1-2 minutes. Add canned tomatoes, pinto beans, bay leaf and water. Cover and bring to a boil. Reduce heat to low and cook until beans are quite soft and soup has become creamy, 1 to 1 ½ hours.

While the soup cooks, make the pesto. Combine ingredients in a food processor and puree until smooth, adding a small amount of water, if needed, to thin the consistency. Adjust seasoning to taste. Do not make the pesto too thin or it will not rest on top of the soup.

When the beans are quite soft, remove a small amount of broth, puree miso and stir in. Simmer soup, uncovered, for 3-4 minutes to activate the enzymes in the miso. Remove bay leaf and discard.

To serve, ladle soup into individual bowls with a dollop of pesto on top. Makes 4-5 servings.

White Bean Soup with Spelt

Beans and grains come together in this creamy soup to create a complete protein, creating the perfect environment to utilize nutrients most efficiently. Laced through with sweet vegetables, this soup is like a symphony of flavors on your tongue.

Extra virgin olive oil
2 cloves fresh garlic, finely minced
1 small yellow onion, diced
sea salt
1 carrot, diced
1 cup diced butternut squash, do not peel
½ cup spelt, rinsed well, soaked for 1 hour, drained well
1 cup cannellini beans, sorted, rinsed well
1 bay leaf
5 cups spring or filtered water
2 teaspoons sweet white miso
3-4 leaves fresh kale, finely minced
½ red bell pepper, roasted over an open flame, peeled, seeded, finely minced

Place a small amount of oil, garlic and onion in a medium soup pot over medium heat. When the onion begins to sizzle, add a pinch of salt and sauté for 2-3 minutes. Stir in carrot and squash, a pinch of salt and sauté for 1-2 minutes. Add spelt, beans, bay leaf and water, cover and bring to a boil. Reduce heat to low and cook until beans and spelt are quite soft, 1 to 1 ½ hours. When the spelt is soft, remove a small amount of broth, dissolve miso and stir it, along with minced greens into soup. Simmer for 3-4 minutes to activate the enzymes in the miso. Remove bay leaf and discard. Serve garnished with roasted pepper. Makes 4-6 servings.

Mixed Bean Potage

We're all obsessed with protein and all that it brings to us . . . or so we think. This simple soup will satisfy all the high-protein lovers fondest wishes for strength and weight management.

Extra virgin olive oil
2-3 cloves fresh garlic, finely minced
1 red onion, finely diced
sea salt
generous pinch crushed red pepper flakes
2-3 stalks celery, large dice
2 carrot, large dice
1 small sweet potato, large dice
½ cup white wine
¼ cup chickpeas, sorted, rinsed well
¼ cup red kidney beans, sorted, rinsed well
¼ cup cannellini beans, sorted, rinsed well
¼ cup green lentils, sorted, rinsed well
1 bay leaf
4 cups spring or filtered water
3-4 sprigs fresh parsley, finely minced

Place about 3 tablespoons oil, the garlic and onion in a medium soup pot over medium heat. When the onions begin to sizzle, add a pinch of sea salt and red pepper flakes and sauté for 1-2 minutes. Stir in celery, carrot and sweet potato, a pinch of salt and sauté for 2-3 minutes. Add white wine and bring to the boil. Stir in beans and bay leaf. Add water, cover and bring to a boil. Reduce heat to low and cook until chickpeas are quite soft, 1 to 1 ½ hours. Remove bay leaf, season to taste with salt and simmer for another 5-7 minutes. Serve garnished with minced parsley. Makes 4-5 servings.

Chickpea and Arugula Soup

Combining the sweet, nutty flavor of chickpeas with the delicate bitter flavor of crisp arugula and you have the most delicious soup. On top of that, this soup is packed with protein and other nutrients and so easy to digest thanks to the greens.

Extra virgin olive oil
2-3 cloves fresh garlic, thinly sliced
1 yellow onion, diced
sea salt

generous pinch crushed red pepper flakes
½ cup white wine
1 carrot, diced
1 cup diced daikon
1 cup diced butternut squash
1 cup chickpeas, sorted, rinsed well
1 bay leaf
4 cups spring or filtered water
2 teaspoons white miso
5-6 stems fresh arugula, rinsed very well, hand shredded

Place a small amount of oil, garlic and onion in a medium soup pot over medium heat. When the onions begin to sizzle, stir in a pinch of salt and the red pepper flakes and sauté for 1-2 minutes. Add white wine and sauté until it reduces, about 2 minutes. Stir in carrot, daikon, squash and a pinch of salt and sauté until shiny with oil. Add chickpeas, bay leaf and water, cover and bring to a boil. Reduce heat to low and simmer until chickpeas are quite soft, 1 to 1 ½ hours. Remove a small amount of broth, dissolve miso and stir into soup. Simmer, uncovered, for 3-4 minutes to activate the enzymes in the miso. Remove bay leaf and discard. Just before serving, stir shredded arugula into soup. Makes 4-5 servings.

Curried Yellow Split Pea Soup

The delicate spiced heat of curry and split peas go together like Romeo and Juliet . . . but it's better than love. The heat of the curry stimulates circulation, enhancing our body's ability to digest efficiently . . . and the protein of the beans gives us the strength we need to feed our bones.

Extra virgin olive oil
2-3 cloves fresh garlic, finely minced
1 small red onion, diced
2/3 teaspoon curry paste
sea salt
1 carrot, diced
2 stalks celery, diced
grated zest of 1 lemon
3-4 okra, diced
1 cup yellow split peas, rinsed very well
4 cups spring or filtered water
1 bay leaf
2-3 spring fresh basil, finely shredded

Place about 3 tablespoons oil, garlic and onion in a soup pot over medium heat. When the onions begin to sizzle, stir in curry paste and a pinch of salt and sauté for 2-3 minutes, to develop the 'heat' of the curry paste. Stir in carrot and celery and a pinch of salt and sauté for 1-2 minutes. Stir in lemon zest and okra, a pinch of salt and sauté for 1 minute. Add peas, water and bay leaf and bring to a boil covered. Reduce heat to low and cook until peas are quite soft, 45 minutes to 1 hour. Remove bay leaf and discard. Season the soup to taste with salt and simmer soup for 7-10 minutes more, stirring occasionally. Serve soup garnished with shredded fresh basil. Makes 4-6 servings.

White Bean and Cabbage Soup with Polenta

Beans and grains work together perfectly, creating a complete protein. The silky texture of the white beans provides the perfect backdrop to the sweet, comforting nature of cabbage, with the energizing nature of corn grits to keep us interested.

Extra virgin olive oil
2-3 cloves fresh garlic, finely minced
1 yellow onion, diced
generous pinch crushed red pepper flakes
sea salt
¼ head green cabbage, finely diced
½ cup yellow corn grits
1 cup cannellini beans, rinsed well
1 bay leaf
5 cups spring or filtered water
3 tablespoons sweet white miso
2-3 sprigs fresh basil, finely shredded

Place about 3 tablespoons oil, garlic and onion in a soup pot over medium heat. When the onions begin to sizzle, add red pepper flakes and a pinch of salt and sauté for 2-3 minutes. Stir in cabbage, a pinch of salt and sauté until cabbage wilts, 3-4 minutes. Add grits, beans, bay leaf and water and bring to a boil covered. Reduce heat to low and cook until beans are soft, 1 to 1 ½ hours. Remove a small amount of broth and puree miso. Stir miso back into soup and simmer for 3-4 minutes to activate the enzymes, taking care not to boil (as this destroys the enzymes in the miso). Remove bay leaf and discard. Serve garnished with fresh basil. Makes 4-6 servings.

Squash and Chickpea Soup

Life isn't as sweet without the bitter . . . at least that's how the saying goes. In this soup, it's pure sweetness. Sautéed onions and winter squash are combined with the delicate sweet taste of chickpeas to create a powerful protein punch.

Avocado oil
1 yellow onion, diced
sea salt
1 medium butternut squash, peeled, seeded, diced
2 cups spring or filtered water
2 cups unsweetened soymilk
1 ½ cooked chickpeas (or canned organic chickpeas)
1 ½ tablespoons sweet white miso
1-2 fresh scallions, thinly sliced on the diagonal

Place about 3 tablespoons oil and the onion in a soup pot over medium heat. When the onions begin to sizzle, add a pinch of salt and sauté for 1-2 minutes. Stir in squash and sauté just until shiny with oil. Add soymilk and water, cover loosely and bring to a boil. Reduce heat to low and cook until squash is tender, about 35 minutes. Transfer soup, by ladles, to a food processor and puree until smooth. Return to pot, place over low heat and stir in chickpeas. Cook for 5 minutes. Remove a small amount of broth and puree miso. Stir into soup and simmer for 3-4 minutes to activate the enzymes, taking care not to boil (boiling will destroy enzymes in miso). Remove bay leaf and discard. Serve garnished with scallions. Makes 4-6 servings.

Thick Vegetable Soup with Fava Beans

A hearty vegetable soup can be a meal in itself, laced through with an abundant amount of seasonal vegetables. We've upped the ante of protein . . . and yummy flavor . . . by stirring in fava beans.

Extra virgin olive oil
2-3 cloves fresh garlic, finely minced
1 red onion, diced
1 small leek, split lengthwise, rinsed free of dirt, diced
sea salt
2-3 stalks celery, diced

2 carrots, diced
¼ head green cabbage, diced
¼ cauliflower, tiny florets
1 small fennel bulb, tops removed, diced
1 cup dry white wine
3 cups spring or filtered water
1 ½ cups fresh or frozen fava beans
1-2 sprigs fresh basil, finely shredded

Place about 3 tablespoons oil, garlic, onion and leek in a medium soup pot over medium heat. When the onions begin to sizzle, add a pinch of salt and sauté until leeks wilt, about 2 minutes. Stir in celery and carrot, a pinch of salt and sauté for 1 minute. Stir in cabbage and cauliflower, a pinch of salt and sauté for 1 minute. Stir in fennel and wine and cook, stirring for 1 minute. Add water, cover and bring to a boil. Reduce heat and cook until vegetables are soft, about 25 minutes. Remove bay leaf and discard. Season with salt to taste and stir in fava beans. Cook for 7-10 minutes more to develop the flavor of the salt. Serve garnished with fresh basil. Makes 4 to 5 servings.

Okra, Tomato and Black-Eyed Pea Soup

Black-eyed peas don't get the attention they deserve. Glossed over as 'southern' in American cuisine, these delicious beans are widely used in Mediterranean cooking. Packed with nutrients like calcium, magnesium, good quality fat and protein, black-eyed peas are a great source of vitality . . . and the stars of this delicious soup. And okra? A rich source of calcium and oh, so yummy in this soup.

Extra virgin olive oil
2-3 cloves fresh garlic, thinly sliced
1 red onion, diced
sea salt
generous pinch crushed red pepper flakes
2-3 stalks celery, diced
2 small zucchini, diced (or 1 large)
8-10 okra, diced
4-5 vine-ripened tomatoes, diced (do not seed or peel)
1 cup black-eyed peas, rinsed very well
1 bay leaf
4 cups spring or filtered water
1 ½ tablespoons sweet white miso
2-3 sprigs fresh parsley, finely minced

Place about 3 tablespoons oil, garlic and red onion in a medium soup pot over medium heat. When the onion begins to sizzle, add a pinch of salt and the red pepper flakes and sauté for 1-2 minutes. Stir in celery, zucchini, a pinch of salt and sauté for 1 minute. Stir in okra and tomatoes, a pinch of salt and sauté for 1 minute. Add beans, bay leaf and water, cover and bring to a boil, covered. Reduce heat to low and cook until beans are soft, about 1 to 1 ½ hours. Remove a small amount of broth and puree miso. Stir into soup and simmer for 3-4 minutes to activate the enzymes, taking care not to boil (boiling destroys the enzymes in the miso). Remove bay leaf and discard. Serve garnished with fresh parsley. Makes 4-6 servings.

Whole Carp Soup

This version of carp soup, a classic macrobiotic vitality enhancer, is a bit of work, but so calcium-rich that it's sure to help build strong bones. Delicious and rich, this is a fish lover's delight . . . . oh, and it makes you big and strong.

Extra virgin olive oil
1/2-inch piece fresh ginger, finely minced
1 red onion, diced
sea salt
1 pound of carrots, fine matchstick pieces
1 pound of burdock, fine matchstick pieces
2 pound carp, cut into 2-inch pieces (have the fish monger remove only the thyroid and the yellow bone. Retain the balance of the fish, even the scales . . .)
1 cup kukicha tea twigs, wrapped in cheesecloth
spring or filtered water
barley miso
3-4 fresh scallions, thinly sliced on the diagonal

Place about 3 tablespoons oil, ginger and onion in a deep pressure cooker over medium heat. When the onion begins to sizzle, add a pinch of salt and sauté for 1-2 minutes. Stir in carrot, a generous pinch of salt and sauté until shiny with oil. Stir in burdock, a generous pinch of salt and sauté until just limp. Add the carp, the wrapped kukicha twigs and add water to generously cover the fish. Seal the lid of the pressure cooker and bring to full pressure. Reduce heat to low and cook for 1 hour. Turn off heat and allow pressure to reduce naturally. Open pressure cooker and test the fish for tenderness. It should be very soft; even the bones should be soft. Remove the kukicha bundle and discard. Using a wooden spoon, break up the fish into small pieces in the soup. Cook the soup for another

45 minutes. Remove about one cup of broth and puree in it, one teaspoon of miso per cup of water added for cooking. Stir into soup and simmer for 3-4 minutes to activate the enzymes, taking care not to boil (boiling destroys the enzymes in the miso). Serve garnished with scallion. Makes 10-12 servings.

Note: Usually, this soup is served in one-cup bowls, five days in a row, freezing the balance in five-serving portions. Repeat this serving method 2 weeks later and 2 weeks after that. Also note that the weight of the carrot and burdock must equal the weight of the carp.

Mexican Black Bean Soup with Tofu Sour Cream

Black beans and hot spice go together like love and marriage. Add to it the minerals, protein, carbohydrates, good quality fats and other nutrients inherent to black beans and you have the perfect relationship of deliciousness and good health. Topped with phytoestrogen-rich tofu sour cream is just the icing on the cake for our bones.

Extra virgin olive oil
2-3 cloves fresh garlic, finely minced
1 red onion, diced
grated zest of 1 lemon
1 dried jalapeno chili, soaked until tender, diced
sea salt
1-2 stalks celery, diced
1 carrot, diced
1 ½ cups canned diced tomatoes
1 cup black turtle beans, rinsed very well
1 bay leaf
4 cups spring or filter water

tofu sour cream:
1 cup silken or soft tofu
sea salt
juice of 1 fresh lemon
2-3 sprigs, fresh cilantro, finely minced

Place about 3 tablespoons oil, garlic, onion, lemon zest and chili in a medium soup pot over medium heat. When the onion begins to sizzle, add a pinch of salt and sauté for 2-3 minutes. Stir in celery and carrot, a pinch of salt and sauté for 1-2 minutes. Stir in tomatoes. Add beans, bay leaf and water, cover and bring to a boil. Reduce heat to low and cook until beans are soft, 1 to 1 ½ hours. When the beans are soft, season the soup to taste with salt. Remove bay leaf and discard.

While the soup cooks, make the tofu sour cream. In a food processor, puree tofu until smooth. Add salt and lemon juice to taste, to simulate the flavor of sour cream.

To serve, ladle soup into individual bowls with a generous dollop of tofu sour cream and a sprinkle of cilantro. Makes 4-5 servings.

Italian Lentil Soup

When I was a kid, I hated my mother's lentil soup, or anything with beans, for that matter. Who knew this simple soup was not only designed to feed my tummy, but to nourish my bones with calcium, protein and perfectly balanced trace minerals?

Extra virgin olive oil
2-3 cloves fresh garlic, finely minced
1 small red onion, diced
sea salt
generous pinch crushed red pepper flakes
2-3 stalks celery, diced
1 carrot, diced
1 16-ounce can diced tomatoes
1 cup green or brown lentils, rinsed very well
4 cups spring or filtered water
1 bay leaf
2-3 sprigs fresh basil, finely shredded

Place about 3 tablespoons oil, garlic and onion in a medium soup pot over medium heat. When the onion begins to sizzle, add a pinch of salt and the crushed red pepper and sauté for 1 minute. Stir in celery and carrot, a pinch of salt and sauté for 1 minute. Stir in tomatoes and bring to a gentle boil. Add lentils, water and bay leaf, cover and bring to a boil. Reduce heat to low and cook until lentils are quite soft, about an hour. Season to taste with salt, remove bay leaf and simmer for 7-10 more minutes to develop flavors. Serve garnished with fresh basil. Makes 4-5 servings.

Miso Soup with Wakame and Vegetables

A staple of whole foods cooking, miso is said to have been given to man by the gods to promote good health and enlightenment. I don't know about that, but miso is rich in friendly bacteria and enzymes that promote intestinal health . . . and good digestion means getting all the nutrients our food has to offer. And the sea plant, wakame is rich in the trace minerals we need for strong blood.

4 cups spring or filtered water
3 inches wakame, soaked until tender, diced
½ yellow onion, thin half moon pieces
½ small carrot, thin half moon pieces
½ cup fresh daikon, thin half moon pieces
4 teaspoons barley or brown rice miso
2 scallions, thinly sliced on the diagonal

Place water in a medium sauce pan with wakame. Bring to a boil. Add onions, carrots and daikon, cover and bring to a boil. Reduce heat to low and cook until vegetables are tender, about 5 minutes. Remove a small amount of broth and puree miso. Stir into soup and simmer for 3-4 minutes to activate the enzymes, taking care not to boil (boiling destroys the enzymes in miso). Serve garnished with fresh scallion. Makes about 4 servings.

Note: When reheating miso soup, take special care not to boil it to insure integrity of the enzymes in the miso.

Fish Chowder

A vegan by choice, I had a lot of reflecting to do when Robert was diagnosed with osteoporosis. Ultimately the foods he needed to regain his health far outweighed my moral life choices, so I developed several fish recipes to give him the nutrients he needed, balanced with lots of vegetables to support digestion and health.

Extra virgin olive oil
2-3 cloves fresh garlic, thinly sliced
1 red onion, diced
sea salt
generous pinch crushed red pepper flakes
2-3 stalks celery, diced
1-2 carrots, diced

1 cup diced butternut squash
½ cup diced daikon
½ cup diced zucchini
1 fresh tomato, diced, do not peel or seed (if out of season, use 8 ounces diced, canned tomatoes)
6 ounces, white meat fish, coarsely chopped, cod, flounder, trout, haddock, monkfish
2 cups spring or filtered water
3 cups plain soymilk
1 bay leaf
5 teaspoons sweet white miso
3-4 sprigs fresh parsley, finely minced

Place about 3 tablespoons oil, garlic and onion in a medium soup pot over medium heat. When the onions begin to sizzle, add a pinch of salt and red pepper flakes and sauté for 1 minute. Stir in celery and carrot, a pinch of salt and sauté for 1 minute. Stir in squash, a pinch of salt and sauté for 1 minute. Stir in daikon, a pinch of salt and sauté for 1 minute. Stir in zucchini and tomato. Top with fish and add water, soymilk and bay leaf. Cover and bring to a boil. Reduce heat to low and cook until fish is quite soft, 30-35 minutes. Remove a small amount of broth and puree miso. Stir into soup and simmer for 3-4 minutes to activate the enzymes in the miso, taking care not to boil (boiling destroys the enzymes in the miso). Serve garnished with fresh parsley. Makes 6-7 servings.

Note: You may freeze this soup in portions for later use.

Hot and Sour Tofu Noodle Soup

Don't let tofu's mild mannered character fool you. This humble soyfood is a powerhouse of nutrition. Packed with phytonutrients, protein and other trace minerals, tofu is a valuable tool in keeping our bones strong.

Light sesame oil
½-inch piece fresh ginger, finely minced
1 small leek, split lengthwise, rinsed free of dirt, thinly sliced
soy sauce
1 tablespoon brown rice syrup
generous pinch crushed red pepper flakes
1-2 stalks celery, very thinly sliced

1 carrot, very fine matchstick pieces
½ cup very fine daikon matchstick pieces
½ brick extra firm tofu, small cubes
4 cups spring or filtered water
3 ounces whole wheat somen noodles, cooked al dente
2 teaspoons kuzu, dissolved in small amount cold water
brown rice vinegar

Heat a small amount of oil in a medium soup pot and sauté ginger and leek, with a pinch of soy sauce, over medium heat. Stir in rice syrup and red pepper flakes. Stir in celery, a splash of soy sauce and sauté for 1 minute. Stir in carrot, a splash of soy sauce and sauté for 1 minute. Stir in daikon, a splash of soy sauce and sauté for 1 minute. Add tofu and water, cover and bring to a boil. Reduce heat to low and simmer until carrots are tender, about 7 minutes. Season to taste with soy sauce and cook for 7 minutes more. Stir in noodles and dissolved kuzu and cook stirring until soup thickens slightly, about 2 minutes. Remove from heat and stir in a generous splash of brown rice vinegar. Makes 4-5 servings.

White Bean and Bitter Greens Soup

The protein in beans can be difficult for some people to digest . . . hence the little poems. But the health benefits of beans are without compare, so what do we do? Combining beans with bitter greens takes out all the guess work. The greens work to aid the body in the efficient assimilation of the protein in beans. And yummy? Just taste this soup.

Extra virgin olive oil
2-3 cloves fresh garlic, thinly sliced
1 red onion, diced
sea salt
generous pinch crushed red pepper flakes
2-3 stalks celery, diced
4-5 vine-ripened tomatoes, diced, do not peel or seed
1 cup white beans, cannellini, navy, great northern, rinsed very well
1 cup dry white wine
3 cups spring or filtered water
1 bay leaf
4 teaspoons sweet white miso
2-3 sprigs fresh parsley, finely minced

Place about 3 tablespoons oil, garlic and red onion in a medium soup pot over medium heat. When the onion begins to sizzle, add a pinch of salt and the red pepper flakes and sauté for 1-2 minutes. Stir in celery, a pinch of salt and sauté for 1-2 minutes. Stir in tomatoes, a pinch of salt and sauté for 1-2 minutes. Add beans, wine, water and bay leaf, cover and bring to a boil. Reduce heat to low and cook until beans are quite soft, about an hour. Remove a small amount of broth and puree miso. Stir into soup and simmer for 3-4 minutes to activate the enzymes, taking care not to boil (boiling destroys the enzymes in the miso). Serve garnished with fresh parsley. Makes 4-5 servings.

Fresh Corn Chowder with Hempseed Pesto

We take nutrient-packed corn and rachet things up by adding avocado oil, creamy soymilk, miso and a richly-flavored hempseed pesto for all the protein and essential fatty acids you might need in one bowl of soup.

Avocado oil
1 yellow onion, diced
sea salt
2-3 stalks celery, diced
1-2 small yellow summer squash, diced
1-2 small zucchini, diced
2 cups fresh/frozen corn kernels
2 cups unsweetened soymilk
2 cups spring or filtered water
4 teaspoons sweet white miso

hempseed pesto:
1 cup loosely packed fresh basil leaves
½ cup pine nuts
1 cup shelled hempseeds
2-3 cloves fresh garlic, finely minced
1/3 cup extra virgin olive oil
1 tablespoon sweet white miso
1 teaspoon brown rice syrup

Place about 3 tablespoons oil and onion in a medium soup pot over medium heat. When the onion begins to sizzle, add a pinch of salt and sauté for 1-2 minutes. Stir in celery, a pinch of salt and sauté for 1 minute. Stir in summer squash and zucchini, a pinch of salt and sauté for 1 minute. Stir in corn, soymilk and water, cover and bring to a boil. Cook until vegetables are soft, about 15 minutes. Remove a small amount of broth and puree miso. Stir into soup and simmer for 3-4 minutes to activate the enzymes, taking care not to boil (boiling destroys the enzymes in miso).

Make the pesto while the soup cooks. Place basil leaves, pine nuts, hempseeds and garlic in a food processor and puree until coarse. Add oil, miso and rice syrup and puree until a thick paste forms.

To serve, ladle soup into individual bowls and top with a generous dollop of pesto. Makes 4-5 servings.

Note: You may have extra pesto. It's brilliant on pasta or spread on bread.

Cannellini, Tomato and Basil Soup

Tomato soup with a protein punch. With the mild flavor of white beans to provide the protein we crave, we're free to spice up the flavors in this delicate, but mighty soup.

Extra virgin olive oil
2-3 cloves fresh garlic, finely minced
1 red onion, diced
sea salt
generous pinch crushed red pepper flakes
2-3 stalks celery, diced
1-2 small zucchini, diced
5-6 vine-ripened tomatoes, diced, do not peel or seed
1 cup cannellini beans, rinsed very well
1 bay leaf
4 cups spring or filtered water
4 teaspoons sweet white miso
3-4 sprigs fresh basil, finely shredded

Place about 3 tablespoons oil, garlic and onion in a medium soup pot over medium heat. When the onion begins to sizzle, add a pinch of salt and red pepper flakes and sauté for 1-2 minutes. Stir in celery and zucchini, a pinch of salt and sauté for 1 minute. Stir in tomatoes, a pinch of salt and sauté for 1 minute. Add beans, bay leaf and water, cover and bring to a boil, covered. Reduce heat to low and cook until beans are quite soft, about an hour. Remove a small amount of broth and puree miso. Stir into soup and simmer for 3-4 minutes to activate the enzymes, taking care not to boil (boiling destroys the enzymes in the miso). Stir in basil and serve. Makes 4-5 servings.

Curried Cauliflower and Red Lentil Dahl

The mild character of cauliflower makes the perfect companion to the spicy heat of curry and together, they help ease the digestion of beans, making this soup a great source of protein that will be easily assimilated by our tender systems and used to our best ability.

Extra virgin olive oil
2-3 cloves fresh garlic, minced
1 yellow onion, diced
sea salt
½-2/3 teaspoon curry powder
2-3 stalks celery, diced
1 carrot, diced
1 cup diced butternut squash
1 cup red lentils, rinsed very well
1 bay leaf
1 cup plain soymilk
3 cups spring or filtered water
¼ cup dry white wine
1-2 sprigs flat leaf parsley, finely minced

Place about 3 tablespoons oil, garlic and onion in a medium soup pot over medium heat. When the onion begins to sizzle, add a pinch of salt and curry powder and sauté for 2-3 minutes to activate the heat of the curry. Stir in celery, a pinch of salt and sauté for 1 minute. Stir in carrot and squash, a pinch of salt and sauté for 1 minute. Add lentils, bay leaf, soymilk, water and wine, cover and bring to a boil. Reduce heat to low and cook until lentils are quite creamy, 45 minutes to 1 hour. Season to taste with salt and cook for another 7-10 minutes. Serve garnished with parsley. Makes 4-5 servings.

Kidney Bean and Corn Chowder

Nothing lightens up bean chowder quite like fresh corn kernels. The bright color and delicate sweet taste add a depth of flavor that makes this chowder sparkle with vitality.

Extra virgin olive oil
1 yellow onion, diced
sea salt
2-3 stalks celery, diced

1 carrot, diced
1 small zucchini, diced
1 yellow summer squash, diced
1 cup canned diced tomatoes
1 cup red kidney beans, rinsed very well
1 bay leaf
2 cups spring or filtered water
2 cups plain soymilk
4 teaspoons sweet white miso
1 cup fresh/frozen corn kernels
2-3 sprigs fresh parsley, finely minced

Place about 3 tablespoons oil and onion in a medium soup pot over medium heat. When the onion begins to sizzle, add a pinch of salt and sauté for 1-2 minutes. Stir in celery, a pinch of salt and sauté for 1 minute. Stir in carrot, a pinch of salt and sauté for 1 minute. Stir in zucchini and yellow squash, a pinch of salt and sauté for 1 minute. Add tomatoes, kidney beans, bay leaf, water and soymilk, cover and bring to a boil. Reduce heat to low and cook until beans are soft, 1 to 1 ½ hours. Stir in corn. Remove a small amount of broth and puree miso. Stir into soup and simmer for 3-4 minutes to activate the enzymes, taking care not to boil (boiling destroys the enzymes in miso). Serve garnished with parsley. Makes 4-5 servings.

Chapter 8

Grains . . . The Core of Strength

I can hear you all now. Grains? Grains? Aren't they carbohydrates? Aren't they a part of the axis of evil in our modern world of protein obsession? Well, hold onto your hats and hear me out before you run from the room screaming.

Whole cereal grains are the foundation of health, the centerpiece food for humanity. So is it any wonder that grain would be an essential factor in your day to day vitality, with our bones as our foundation of strength?

We all know that fiber, like that in whole grains, is an important factor in the prevention of colon cancer, diverticulitis, ulcers, appendicitis, hemorrhoids and many other digestive disorders, but we really don't associate digestive function with strong bones. Here's a news flash. The quality of nutrients taken into the body, along with how well they are assimilated, is responsible for the nourishment—or starvation of the living tissue that makes up our bones (and the rest of us). Therefore, foods that strengthen digestion and stimulate circulation are essential for a strong, dense bones.

The fiber in whole grains is even more brilliant, though. Not only responsible for digestive function, the soluble fiber found in grain, especially brown rice and oats, has been found to lower cholesterol, reducing the risk of coronary diseases and prevent blockages in capillaries that supply nutrients to all the cells in our bodies . . . including, yes our bones.

Because of their structure, the complex carbohydrates in whole grains are also essential to healthy bones. Since they break down slowly, they are not absorbed into the bloodstream until they reach the villi in the small intestine. So unlike simple sugars that are rapidly absorbed, complex sugars will strengthen the ability of the digestive system to circulate nutrients to the body.

Whole grains also contain perfectly balanced nutrients—an average of seven to one—the ratio of minerals to protein is about one to seven; protein to carbohydrate is also one to seven, making grain the ideal food to support and nourish smooth, even growth cycles of our bones.

But whole grains do even more. The fiber, complex sugars, minerals, protein and B-vitamins so abundant in then are key to our bones' health and strength. The intestines are responsible for regulating moisture in the body as well as for influencing the quality of the blood that will nourish all of our organs, determining their health and function. If the intestines are efficiently nourished, their work influences the creation of strong, balanced blood, which in turn circulates through our other organ systems, supporting the creation of new bone tissue.

So go to the kitchen and cook a pot of rice—or quinoa, or amaranth or barley or whole wheat pasta . . . and stand tall with a strong, dense skeleton.

Tomato-Laced Quinoa

This ancient grain, known by the Aztecs as the 'mother seed,' is a powerhouse of nutrients . . . amino acids in a near perfect balance, more protein than any other cereal grain and lysine for digestion . . . and did I mention how delicious it is?

Extra virgin olive oil
1 teaspoon red chili paste
sea salt
black pepper
½ red onion, finely diced
2 vine-ripened tomatoes, diced, do not peel or seed
1 cup quinoa, rinsed very well
2 cups spring or filtered water
2-3 sprigs fresh basil, shredded

Place about 2 tablespoons oil in a skillet over medium heat. When the oil is hot, add the chili paste and sauté until well-blended into the oil. Add a pinch of salt and black pepper and add onion. Sauté for 2-3 minutes. Stir in tomatoes, add a pinch of salt and sauté for 2-3 minutes, until tomatoes are coated with oil. Spread veggies evenly on the bottom of the skillet and cover. Reduce heat to low and cook until tomatoes are lightly browned and wilted, 15-20 minutes.

Combine quinoa and water in a sauce pan and bring to a boil. Add a light seasoning of salt, cover and reduce heat to low. Cook until water is absorbed into the grain and the quinoa has opened up, about 20-25 minutes. Fluff with a fork.

To serve, simply stir braised tomatoes and fresh basil into quinoa and serve immediately. Makes 3-4 servings.

Spicy Baked Quinoa

Baked grain can be so incredibly satisfying and strengthening. And with quinoa's protein level, this baked dish turns your bones into Superman!

Extra virgin olive oil
1-2 cloves fresh garlic, finely minced
1 red onion, diced
sea salt
generous pinch crushed red pepper flakes
generous pinch saffron, ground between fingertips
6-8 button mushrooms, brushed free of dirt, thinly sliced
1 carrot, diced
½ cup diced daikon
½ cup dry white wine
1 cup quinoa, rinsed very well
2 cups spring or filtered water
2-3 sprigs fresh parsley, finely minced
juice of ½ lemon

Preheat oven to 350o and lightly oil a 10-inch glass baking dish.

Place about 2 tablespoons oil, garlic and onion in a skillet over medium heat. When the onions begin to sizzle, add a pinch of salt, red pepper flakes, saffron and sauté for 1-2 minutes. Stir in mushrooms, a pinch of salt and sauté for 2-3 minutes. Stir in carrot and daikon, a pinch of salt and sauté for 1-2 minutes. Season lightly with salt and sauté for 1-2 minutes more.

Transfer vegetables to prepared baking dish and top with quinoa and water. Cover tightly with foil and bake for 25-30 minutes. Remove cover, stir gently and return to oven to dry out any remaining liquid and to brown the edges. Stir in parsley and lemon juice and serve immediately. Makes 3-4 servings.

Quinoa-Stuffed Peppers

As whole grains go, quinoa is one of the best for our bones. Easy to digest and packed with protein, quinoa's nutty flavor makes for a great side dish . . . or main course, like this one.

Extra virgin olive oil
1-2 cloves fresh garlic, finely minced
½ red onion, finely diced

sea salt
generous pinch crushed red pepper flakes
1 stalk celery, finely diced
1 carrot, finely diced
½ cup quinoa, rinsed very well
1 cup spring or filtered water
2 red bell peppers, cored and seeded, left whole

tomato sauce:
extra virgin olive oil
1 clove fresh garlic, finely minced
½ red onion, finely diced
sea salt
1, 10-ounce can diced tomatoes
2 sprigs fresh basil, finely shredded
Preheat oven to 350o.

Place a small amount of oil, garlic and onion in a skillet over medium heat. When the onions begin to sizzle, add a pinch of salt and sauté for 1 minute. Stir in red pepper flakes and celery, a pinch of salt and sauté for 1 minute. Add carrot, a pinch of salt and sauté for 1 minute. Stir in quinoa, water and a pinch of salt. Cover and bring to a boil, reduce heat to low and cook until liquid is absorbed and the grain opens, about 25 minutes.

While the quinoa cooks, make the sauce. Place a small amount of oil, garlic and onion in a sauce pan over medium heat. When the onions begin to sizzle, add a pinch of salt and sauté for 1 minute. Stir in tomatoes, season lightly with salt and cook, uncovered, over medium-low heat for 15-20 minutes. Season to taste with salt and stir in basil. Cook for 5 minutes more.

Stir the quinoa to fluff and stuff into each hollowed out pepper, filling abundantly. Stand in a small, shallow baking dish. Spoon tomato sauce over each pepper, covering them, allowing it to spill into the pan. Cover tightly with foil and bake for 25 minutes. Remove the foil and return to the oven for 10 minutes more. Serve immediately. Makes 2-4 servings.

Quinoa Salad with Almonds

Quick to cook, yummy, loaded with protein and other nutrients vital to our bones, quinoa is truly the grain of champions. This salad is just brilliant, richly flavored and satisfying.

Extra virgin olive oil
1-2 cloves fresh garlic, finely diced
½ red onion, finely diced
sea salt
1 stalk celery, finely diced
1 carrot, finely diced
1/3 cup finely diced fresh daikon
2 teaspoons brown rice syrup
1 cup quinoa, rinsed very well
2 cups spring or filtered water
2-3 sprigs fresh cilantro, finely minced
½ cup slivered almonds, lightly pan-toasted
juice of 1 lemon

Place about 3 tablespoons oil, garlic and onion in a skillet over medium heat. When the onions begin to sizzle, add a pinch of salt and sauté for 1 minute. Stir in celery and a pinch of salt and sauté for 1 minute. Stir in carrot and daikon, a pinch of salt and sauté for 1 minute. Add brown rice syrup, stirring until it melts into the veggies. Add quinoa, water and a pinch of salt. Cover and bring to a boil. Reduce heat to low and cook until all liquid is absorbed and the grain opens, about 25 minutes. Remove from heat and stir in cilantro, almonds and lemon juice. Serve immediately. Makes 3-4 servings.

Corn Cakes with Black Beans and Squash

This satisfying main course is a great way to combine beans and grain into a complete protein . . . perfect for our bones . . . and the rest of us, by the way.

Extra virgin olive oil
1-2 cloves fresh garlic, finely minced
1 small yellow onion, diced
sea salt
generous pinch crushed red pepper flakes
1 stalk celery, finely diced
1 cup finely diced butternut squash
½ cup fresh/frozen corn kernels
2-3 fresh scallions, finely minced
1 cup cooked black turtle beans, half mashed
½ cup dry white wine
½ cup extra firm tofu, coarsely crumbled

2-3 sprigs fresh parsley, finely minced
yellow cornmeal

Place about 2 tablespoons oil, garlic and onion in a skillet over medium heat. When the onions begin to sizzle, add a pinch of salt, crushed red pepper flakes and sauté for 1-2 minutes. Add celery, a pinch of salt and sauté for 1 minute. Add corn and scallions, a pinch of salt and sauté for 1 minute. Stir in black beans, wine and season lightly with salt. Cook, uncovered until the wine absorbed, about 10 minutes. Transfer to a mixing bowl and allow to cool to room temperature.

When the mixture has cooled enough to handle, mix in the tofu and parsley, using your hands to incorporate the ingredients. The mixture should be stiff enough to form into patties (if it's too thin, simply mix in some cornmeal to create a stiffer consistency). Form into patties and dredge in cornmeal on both sides. Set aside.

Pour about ¼ inch of oil in a skillet and heat it through on medium-low heat (to ensure that the oil is really hot). Carefully lay patties in oil and cook until lightly browned. Turn the patties and brown on the other side, about 3 minutes each side. Transfer to a platter lined with paper towel to drain. Repeat the frying process with remaining patties.

To serve, place patties on a bed of greens and dress with olive oil and vinegar and a dollop of salsa or serve more conventionally on whole grain buns . . . as burgers, with all the fixings. Makes 3-4 patties.

Almond Rice

Buttery and rich, almond rice feels like a special occasion treat. In fact, it doesn't get easier than this dish. And good for your bones? A complete protein, with rich flavor and lots of nutrients including omega-3, almond rice is a treat you'll want to enjoy often.

1/3 cup almonds
1 cup short grain brown rice, rinsed well, soaked for at least 1 hour
1 ½ cups spring or filtered water
pinch sea salt

Bring a small pot of water to a boil. Drop almonds into the hot water and boil for 3-4 minutes. Drain and cool until you can handle the nuts. Simply slip the skins off the nuts, discard the skins and set almonds aside.

Place rice, almonds and water in a pressure cooker and bring to a boil, loosely covered. Add a pinch of salt and seal the lid. Bring to full pressure, reduce heat to low and cook for 25 minutes. Then turn off the heat and allow the pot to stand, undisturbed for another 25 minutes. Open the lid, stir gently and transfer rice to a serving bowl. Makes 3-4 servings.

Creamy Millet Breakfast Porridge with Almonds, Tofu and Hempseeds

Talk about getting off to a great start . . . this breakfast has a great balance of carbs and protein and will really rev your engines for the day.

½ cup yellow millet, rinsed well
½ cup slivered almonds
½ yellow onion, diced
¼ cup fresh/frozen corn kernels
½ brick extra firm tofu, small cubes
2 ½ cups spring or filtered water
sea salt
3 tablespoons shelled hempseeds
2-3 sprigs fresh parsley, finely minced

Place millet, almonds, onion, corn, tofu and water in a heavy sauce pan and bring to a boil, loosely covered. Add a generous pinch of salt, cover and cook over low heat until all liquid is absorbed and the millet is soft and creamy, about 30 minutes.

While the millet cooks, heat a small skillet and pan toast the hempseeds, over medium-low heat until fragrant, about 2 minutes. Transfer to a small bowl.

When the millet is ready, remove from heat and stir in parsley. Serve with toasted hempseeds on the side. Makes 3-4 servings.

Oat, Dulse and Hempseed Crackers

These crackers have a great crunchy texture and are deliciously strongly flavored. And while great for dipping or serving with soup, they also pack a nutritional punch . . . dulse is rich in the magnesium and potassium we so desperately need and then there are the hempseeds . . . not only yummy, but perfectly balanced nutrition for our bones.

1 cup whole wheat pastry flour
½ cup oat flour*
½ teaspoon sea salt

1 teaspoon baking powder
2 tablespoons dulse, ground into a fine powder
2 tablespoons shelled hempseeds
¼ cup extra virgin olive oil spring or filtered water

Preheat oven to 375o.

Combine all dry ingredients in a mixing bowl and whisk to combine. Cut in oil (with a fork or pastry cutter) to form the texture of wet sand. Slowly add water to achieve a stiff consistency. Roll crackers out on a dry work surface as thinly and evenly as you can. Cut into 1-inch squares and transfer to a parchment-lined baking sheet. Bake on the center rack until edges are lightly browned and crackers are very firm, about 15 minutes. Remove from oven and allow to cool on rack. Cool completely and store in an airtight container. Makes 3-4 servings.

Note: If the crackers get soft after storing, simply place in a 300o oven for 4-5 minutes to re-crisp.

*Make oat flour by grinding oats in a food processor until they become a powdery flour.

Pasta with Spicy Lentil Sauce

Hearty, hot and spicy are the perfect words to sum up this main course. A great source of protein, lentils are also rich in B vitamins, thiamine, folic acid, magnesium and potassium . . . they may be humble, little beans, but they nourish us to the bone.

Extra virgin olive oil
2-3 cloves fresh garlic, finely minced
1 red onion, diced
sea salt
½ dried chili, finely minced, seeds included
1 cup green or brown lentils
1 bay leaf
4 cups spring or filtered water
10 ounces whole wheat penne
1 vine ripened tomato, diced, do not seed or peel
2-3 sprigs fresh basil, finely shredded

Place about 3 tablespoons oil, garlic and onion in a deep sauce pan over medium heat. When the onions begin to sizzle, add a pinch of salt, dried chili and sauté for 1-2 minutes. Add lentils, bay leaf and water. Bring to a boil, cover and reduce heat to low. Cook until lentils are quite soft, about 1 hour.

Drain lentils, reserving cooking liquid. Transfer, by ladles, to a food mill and puree until smooth. Return pureed lentils to pot and slowly stir in cooking liquid to create a thick sauce. Place over low heat, season to taste with salt and cook for 7-10 minutes more.

When the lentils are nearly ready, bring a pot of water to a boil and cook pasta al dente, 8-10 minutes. Drain, but do not rinse. Transfer to a mixing bowl. Immediately toss pasta with cooked lentil sauce, diced tomatoes and basil. Spoon onto a serving platter and drizzle with a fruity olive oil to finish the dish. Makes 3-4 servings.

Cold Sesame Noodles with Broccoli

There is nothing quite like chilled noodles with a creamy, rich sesame sauce . . . so sensual and satisfying. And the best part? Sesame tahini is a fabulous source of useable calcium and adding crisp, fresh broccoli to the dish brings folic acid, vitamin C, magnesium and other trace minerals essential to bone health.

sesame sauce
1 cup sesame tahini
1 teaspoon light sesame oil
2 teaspoons soy sauce
2 teaspoons brown rice syrup
pinch crushed red pepper flakes
juice of 1/2 fresh lemon
2-3 sprigs fresh parsley, finely minced
1-2 stalks fresh broccoli, small florets
8 ounces whole wheat udon noodles

Prepare the sauce by mixing ingredients together. Slowly add water, whisking to create a creamy, thick consistency (do not make the sauce too thin or it will not hold to pasta). Chill sauce completely.

Bring a pot of water to a boil. Cook broccoli until crisp tender, about 3 minutes. Drain well and set aside. In the same water, cook udon noodles al dente, about 12 minutes. Drain and rinse very well and transfer to a mixing bowl.

Loosen sauce with a whisk, adding water if necessary. Mix noodles with sesame sauce. Spoon onto a serving platter, arrange broccoli around the rim and serve immediately. Makes 3-4 servings.

Soba in Dashi with Tofu and Vegetable Tempura

Dashi is a traditional Japanese broth used as the foundation for many dishes. This version, packs a protein punch, is rich in trace minerals and is coupled with good quality fats so all the nutrients in this satisfying dish reach your bones.

light olive or avocado oil
½ brick extra firm tofu
1 red onion, thick half moon slices
1 carrot, thin diagonal slices
6-8 button mushrooms, brushed free of dirt, left whole
2 stalks broccoli, small florets
8 ounces soba noodles
1-2 fresh scallions, thinly sliced on the diagonal

dashi:
3 cups spring or filtered water
2 tablespoons soy sauce
4-5 thin slices fresh ginger
3-inch piece kombu
1 teaspoon bonito flakes* (optional)

tempura batter:
1 cup whole wheat pastry flour
½ cup semolina flour
pinch sea salt
1 teaspoon baking powder
2 teaspoons kuzu, dissolved in small amount cold water
1 bottle dark beer (or sparkling water)

Make the dashi by combining all ingredients in a sauce pan a cooking, covered, over medium-low heat for 15 minutes. Strain broth, removing ginger, kombu and bonito flakes. Place over very low heat, covered, while preparing the rest of the dish.

Make the tempura batter by whisking together dry ingredients. Mix in kuzu and enough beer to create a batter that is the consistency of pancake batter. Set aside for 10 minutes.

Place 3 inches of oil in a deep pot over medium-low heat. Heat oil through to ensure even frying; this could take 10 minutes. You will know the oil is hot enough when patterns form on the bottom of the pot. Raise the heat to high.

Dip tofu cubes in the batter and carefully drop into oil, frying until golden, about 2 minutes. Strain out and drain on paper. Batter and fry remaining vegetables in small batches, draining on paper.

While frying, bring a pot of water to a boil and cook soba al dente, about 12 minutes. Drain and rinse very well.

To serve, place noodles in 4 individual bowls. Spoon dashi over top, mound tempura vegetables and tofu on each bowl and garnish with scallions. Makes 4 main course servings.

* *Bonito flakes are dried tuna flakes and can be found in Asian markets and natural foods stores.*

Amaranth with Apricots

An ancient grain, amaranth is almost as powerfully nutritious as quinoa. Its silky, smooth texture and nutty flavor are matched by its nutritional profile . . . essential amino acids in near perfect balance, rich in protein and trace minerals. Coupled with vitamin C-rich apricots and you have the perfect breakfast grain.

2 cups spring or filtered water
1 cup amaranth, rinsed very well (using a very fine strainer)
6 dried apricots, coarsely chopped
pinch sea salt
shelled hempseeds, lightly pan toasted

Bring water to a boil and whisk in amaranth. Reduce heat to low, stir in apricots and salt, cover and cook until amaranth is creamy, 15-20 minutes. Stir gently and serve immediately garnished with hempseeds. Makes 3-4 servings.

Amaranth and Fresh Corn

Another amaranth favorite in our house. Adding the sweet flavor of fresh corn (not to mention its additional nutrition punch), makes for the perfect summer whole grain side dish.

2 cups spring or filtered water
1 cup amaranth, rinsed very well (using a very fine strainer)

½ cup fresh corn kernels (use organic frozen if fresh is not available)
pinch sea salt
2-3 sprigs fresh parsley, finely minced

Bring water to a boil and whisk in amaranth. Reduce heat to low and stir in corn and salt. Cover and cook until amaranth is creamy, 15-20 minutes. Stir in parsley and serve immediately. Makes 3-4 servings.

Avocado and Pickled Cucumber Nori Rolls

Not just any nori rolls, these. Rich in the essential fatty acid, omega-3 . . . from both the hempseeds and avocado, this richly flavored starter course is a wonderful addition to any buffet table. And you need not tell everyone how good they are for them . . . just let them think they're good!

1 small cucumber, sliced into thin spear
juice of 1 lemon
1 teaspoon soy sauce
2 cups cooked short grain brown rice
¼ cup shelled hempseeds
2 ripe avocados, flesh scooped out whole, thinly sliced
2-3 sheets toasted sushi nori

dipping sauce:
1 cup spring or filtered water
2 teaspoons soy sauce
juice of ½ lemon
scant pinch crushed red pepper flakes

Place cucumbers in a small bowl and add lemon juice and soy sauce. Toss cucumber spears gently in the bowl to coat. Set aside to marinate for 10 minutes.

Mix rice and hempseeds together until seeds are incorporated throughout the rice. Slice avocados and set aside.

Lay a sheet of nori, lengthwise, on a bamboo sushi mat or kitchen towel. With moist hands, press rice firmly onto the nori, about ¼-inch thick, covering the nori end to end, but leaving about ½-inch nori exposed on the edges furthest from and closest to you. Lay cucumber spears on the rice, end to end, near the edge closest to you. Lay avocado slices on top of the cucumber spears.

Using the mat as a guide, wrap the nori around the rice and filling, pressing and rolling jelly-roll style, creating a firm cylinder. Lay the nori roll, seam side down on a dry surface and repeat with remaining ingredients, making 3 nori rolls.

Make the dipping sauce by simply whisking ingredients together, adjusting seasoning to your taste.

Wet the blade of a sharp knife and slice each nori roll into 8 equal pieces. Arrange them, cut side up, on a platter and serve with the dipping sauce. Makes 4-5 servings.

Sesame Rice Sticks

Richly-flavored, whole grain-based, this side dish has everything going for it. With the complex carbohydrates of brown rice to keep you nourished, coupled with the calcium-rich and nutty flavors of sesame seeds . . . you would think that was enough . . . but wait . . . we pan fry these for added richness and better assimilation of the nutrients.

2 cups cooked short or medium grain brown rice
½ cup tan sesame seeds
avocado or light olive oil, for frying

dipping sauce:
1 cup spring or filtered water
2 teaspoons soy sauce
1 teaspoon brown rice vinegar
½ teaspoon powdered ginger
1-2 small shallots, finely minced
1-2 cloves fresh garlic, finely minced

With wet hands, form the rice into firm spears, measuring 3 inches long and ½ inch thick. Dredge in sesame seeds, covering each spear completely. Set aside.

Heat ¼-inch oil in a deep skillet over medium heat. When the oil is hot (you will know the oil is hot when you see patterns forming, called 'dancing'), begin frying rice sticks. Fry a few at a time, until golden, turning gently to ensure even browning. Drain on paper and fry the remainder of the sticks.

Mix the dipping sauce, by whisking ingredients together and adjusting the seasoning to your taste.

Arrange rice sticks on a platter with dipping sauce on the side. Makes 4-5 servings.

Chapter 9

Beans . . . Real Protein for Real People

There has never been a time quite like this . . . in my opinion. Our obsession with protein and dieting is matched only by the dismal results we see. With all the high protein diet plans out there, all the accompanying saturated fat and cholesterol, are we really seeing a thinner America? Hardly. What's the answer? Well, that's another book, but in a word, choosing protein from plant sources will be healthier for our lives . . . and bones. All these high protein plans spell certain disaster for our poor bones as they leach essential minerals and nutrients from our skeletons. Protein from plants? Yep . . . beans.

Beans, simple, humble beans? The stuff of strong bones? Most of us think of beans as—at best, musical and at worst, taking too long to cook, with little pay-off in terms of flavor. In truth, beans are powerhouses of nutrition—the perfect food for creating strength and stamina, without saturated fats to gum up the works. When properly prepared, beans nourish us deeply and deliciously, keeping us . . . and our bones . . . sated and strong.

Protein from plant sources, dismissed in conventional nutrition as not 'complete' is the best source of protein overall. Protein is present in all foods, except fruit, but is especially abundant in beans, bean products and seeds. Plants are the original source of protein on earth. After all, cows eat grass . . . so it makes perfect sense to go right to the source, as it were, for the purest form of protein.

There is only good news about beans and bean products. Rich in protein, they also contain complex carbohydrates, fat, fiber, folic acid and phytochemicals. Plant proteins are less perishable, lower in saturated fatty acids than animal flesh, making them better for our health. The only bad news? When improperly cooked, beans will, in fact, cause people to make up those songs about your beans, but don't worry, we'll get to that.

It's really simple. In order for us to feel our best, we need to feel strong and clear-minded. You will not feel that way eating a diet rich in saturated fats, heavy proteins and here's why. We're all calcium crazy, right? Come on, admit it . . . you worry. When we ingest large quantities of dense protein (like animals), there's one compound in the blood that steps up to the plate to aid the body in assimilating this un-natural protein . . . and it's called serum calcium. It gets better.

When the serum calcium is depleted from continued ingestion of meat and dairy products, precious calcium is leached from our bones to continue the work. Now do you see why we need to supplement calcium? Do you get it? Pass on that steak, chicken, turkey, ice cream and omelet, thank you very much . . . for your bones sake. Your best bet for maintaining vitality, and that includes strong bones, is to avoid animal flesh, using it only as individually needed for strength, and to rely on plant protein for your daily dose of endurance.

You are not doomed to a life of lentils, however—splendid as they are. The choices available to us are as varied as they are delicious, including black turtle beans, azuki beans, kidney beans, split peas, fava, white navy beans, cannellini, cranberry beans, chickpeas and yes, red, green, brown or black lentils—to name just a few. And it doesn't end there.

Along with beans, there are bean by-products. Easy to prepare and requiring less cooking time, tofu and tempeh are most popular and are part of the magical soy category that enchant us so. Soybeans—and thereby soyfoods—are rich in protein, contain a heart-nourishing oil containing some omega-3 fatty acids, contain isoflavones, phytochemicals with hormone-like effects that protect both men and women from certain forms of cancer, when eaten in moderate amounts. Whole soybeans can be tough on our tender tummies, so the brilliant Asian culture discovered many ways to process them, so we may enjoy the many benefits of these wonderful beans. From miso, soy sauce and tamari, soy milk, tofu and tempeh, freshly picked and lightly cooked, soybeans are as delicious as they are beneficial to our vitality.

Convinced to add beans to your diet? Still worried about the musical accompaniment that seems inevitable with them? Follow these simple steps to delicious, silent bean dishes.

1). Rinse dried beans well, soak for about an hour and before cooking, drain them and discard the soaking water. You can skip the soaking process altogether, if you like. It doesn't affect cooking time and the flavor of the cooked dish is actually the richer for lack of soaking. Cooking beans in fresh water eliminates many intestinal difficulties.

2). Bring the beans to a boil over medium heat, uncovered, allowing any bubbles to cook away, rather than lodge in you. Boil them for about five minutes before covering.

3). Finally, add a bay leaf or a small piece of kombu (sea plant) to the water, from the beginning of cooking. Both of these ingredients contain compounds that aid the body in breaking down the protein and fat that can cause digestive struggles with high fiber beans.

4). If using canned beans, rinse them very well before use. The water in the can has become stale and can cause mild stomach upset.

So make no bones about it (you had to know that joke was coming). Whether you choose lentils, cannellini, split peas, black turtle, azuki or black-eyed peas, beans may appear to be humble food, but they are nothing short of the core of our strength.

Pinto Bean Green Rolls

Picture crisp greens wrapped around a richly flavored, slightly spicy bean filling. Sound yummy? It is . . . and loaded with bone-building nutrients, from protein to calcium to folic acid.

green rolls:
6-8 Chinese cabbage, rinsed well, left whole
6-8 collard green leaves, rinsed well, left whole

pinto bean filling:
extra virgin olive oil
1-2 cloves fresh garlic, finely minced
½ red onion, finely diced
sea salt
generous pinch crushed red pepper flakes
1 stalk celery, finely diced
1 small carrot, finely diced
1 vine ripened tomato, finely diced, do not peel or seed
1 cup cooked pinto beans
½ cup dry white wine
2-3 sprigs fresh basil, finely minced

Bring a pot of water to a boil and cook Chinese cabbage leaves until crisp tender, about 2 minutes. Drain and lay flat. In the same water, cook collard leaves until crisp tender, about 2 minutes. Drain and lay flat. Set greens aside to cool while making the filling.

Place about 2 tablespoons oil, garlic and onion in a deep skillet over medium heat. When the onions begin to sizzle, add a pinch of salt and red pepper flakes and sauté for 1 minute. Add celery, a pinch of salt and sauté for 1 minute. Add carrot, a pinch of salt and sauté for 1 minute. Add tomato, beans and white wine, season to taste with salt, cover, reduce heat to low and cook until liquid is absorbed into the beans and the filling is soft and creamy, about 20 minutes. Transfer to a serving bowl to cool.

To assemble the rolls, lay 2 collard leaves on a dry work surface. Lay 2 cabbage leaves on top of the collards. Spoon one quarter of the filling onto the center of the leaves. Pull up the side of the leaves and roll them into spring-roll style shapes. Lay, seam side down to seal. Repeat with remaining ingredients to create 4 rolls.

To serve, slice the rolls in half, on the diagonal, creating 8 equal pieces. Arrange, cut side up, on a platter and serve warm. Makes 4 servings.

Black Bean Stuffed Chayote Squash

The mild-mannered character of this tender squash creates the perfect backdrop for the spicy nature of the filling. The protein of the beans for strength, spice to stimulate circulation, sweet squash to relax us . . . the perfect dish, I'd say.

Extra virgin olive oil
2-3 cloves fresh garlic, finely minced
1 small red onion, diced
sea salt
½ dried chili, finely minced
1-2 stalks celery, diced
1 small carrot, diced
½ cup fresh/frozen corn kernels
1 vine ripened tomato, diced, do not peel or seed
1 cup cooked black beans
½ cup dry white wine
2 chayote squash, halved, seeded

Place about 2 tablespoons oil, garlic and onion in a deep skillet over medium heat. When the onions begin to sizzle, add a pinch of salt, the chili and sauté for 1-2 minutes. Add celery, a pinch of salt and sauté for 1-2 minutes. Add carrot and corn, a pinch of salt and sauté for 1-2 minutes. Add tomatoes, a pinch of salt and sauté for 1 minute. Finally, stir in beans and wine and bring to a boil. Season to taste with salt, cover and reduce heat to low. Cook until all liquid is absorbed into the beans, about 15 minutes.

Preheat oven to 350o. Lightly oil the squash halves. Spoon bean filling abundantly into each squash opening and arrange them tightly in a baking dish. Add about ¼ inch water to the baking dish. Cover tightly and bake until squash is tender, about 25-30 minutes.

To serve, arrange squash on a serving platter and if you have any filling left, mound it on the platter with the stuffed squash. Makes 4 servings.

White Beans with Fresh Tomato and Basil Sauce

There is nothing in the world quite like this combination (okay, that's dramatic, but you get the idea). White beans are rich sources of protein and trace minerals needed for strong bones, but with a mild character that is just perfect for a spicy, nutrient-packed tomato sauce, with plenty of basil to ensure that you digest all the nutrition.

1 cup cannellini beans, rinsed very well
3 cups spring or filtered water
1 bay leaf

sauce:
extra virgin olive oil
2-3 cloves fresh garlic, finely minced
½ red onion, diced
sea salt
generous pinch crushed red pepper flakes
6-7 vine-ripened tomatoes, diced, do not peel or seed
2/3 cup dry white wine
3-4 sprigs fresh basil, leaves removed from stems, shredded
4-5 oil-cured black olives, pitted, coarsely chopped

Place beans, water and bay leaf in a heavy pot over medium heat. Bring to a boil, uncovered and boil for 5 minutes. Cover, reduce heat to low and cool until beans are tender, about an hour. Drain liquid away so beans do not get too soft.

While the beans cook, prepare the sauce. Place about 2 tablespoons oil, garlic and onion in a deep skillet over medium heat. When the onions begin to sizzle, add a pinch of salt and the red pepper flakes and sauté for 2-3 minutes. Stir in tomatoes and wine and bring to a boil.

Cover and reduce heat to low and cook for 15 minutes. Season lightly with salt and simmer for another 5 minutes.

Stir in cooked beans, basil and olives and cook for 5 minutes. Transfer to a serving platter and serve immediately. Makes 3-4 servings.

Chickpeas with Tomatoes and Basil over Pasta

One concern for vegetarians is getting enough complete protein. One of the ways to do that is to create a classic combination like grains and beans or pasta and beans. In this dish, we create not only complete protein, but complete satisfaction.

Extra virgin olive oil
1-2 cloves fresh garlic, thinly sliced
1 red onion, thin half moon slices
sea salt
1-2 stalks celery, thin diagonal slices
1 carrot, fine matchstick pieces
3-4 vine-ripened tomatoes, thin half moon slices, do not peel or seed
1 cup cooked chickpeas
1 cup dry white wine
2-3 sprigs fresh parsley, finely minced
1 pound orecchiette

Place about 3 tablespoons oil, garlic and onion in a deep skillet over medium heat. When the onions begin to sizzle, add a pinch of salt and sauté for 2-3 minutes. Add celery, a pinch of salt and sauté for 1-2 minutes. Add carrot, a pinch of salt and sauté for 1-2 minutes. Stir in tomatoes, chickpeas, a pinch of salt and wine and bring to a boil. Cover and reduce heat to low. Cook until chickpeas are quite soft, about 15 minutes. Season to taste with salt and cook, uncovered, until the sauce thickens slightly, about 5 minutes.

While the sauce cooks, bring a pot of water to a boil. Add a pinch of salt and a drizzle of oil. Cook pasta al dente, 9-10 minutes. Drain, but do not rinse. Stir pasta and parsley into chickpea mixture and stir well to combine. Transfer to a serving platter and serve immediately. Makes 4-5 servings.

Split Pea Hummus

A yummy twist on a classic Middle Eastern recipe . . . this version of hummus is creamy, richly flavored and delightfully different . . . but with the same nutrient-dense qualities we love so much in hummus.

1 cup green split peas, rinsed very well
2 ½ cups spring or filtered water
1 bay leaf
¼ cup extra virgin olive oil
¼ cup sesame tahini
sea salt
2-3 cloves fresh garlic, very finely minced
2 teaspoons brown rice syrup or honey
generous pinch crushed red pepper flakes
juice of 1/2 lemon

Place split peas, water and bay leaf in a heavy pot and bring to a boil, uncovered and boil for 5 minutes. Cover, reduce heat to low and cook until split peas are quite soft, about 1 hour.

Transfer the peas to a food processor, add remaining ingredients and puree until smooth. Adjust seasonings to your taste.

Serve with organic corn chips, pita bread, whole grain toast points or celery and carrot sticks. Makes 4-5 servings.

White Beans and Cabbage

This dish may look mild-mannered, but it's packed with protein, antioxidants and trace minerals to keep our bones strong and dense. Mother Nature is brilliant in her ability to keep us healthy. It's all about balance.

Extra virgin olive oil
1-2 cloves fresh garlic, finely minced
1 small yellow onion, diced
sea salt
1-2 stalks celery, diced
grated zest of 1 lemon
1 cup cannellini beans, rinsed very well
1 cup dry white wine
1 bay leaf
2 cups spring or filtered water
¼ head green cabbage, diced
juice of ½ lemon

Place about 2 tablespoons oil, garlic and onion in a heavy sauce pan over medium heat. When the onions begin to sizzle, add a pinch of salt and sauté for 2-3 minutes. Stir in celery and lemon zest, a pinch of salt and sauté for 1-2 minutes. Spread vegetables over the bottom of the pan and top with beans. Add wine and bring to a boil, uncovered. Add bay leaf and water and return to the boil, uncovered. Cover and reduce heat to low and cook until beans are tender, about 50 minutes. Top beans with cabbage and season lightly with salt, cover and cook until cabbage is tender, 7-10 minutes. Remove cover and continue cooking until any remaining liquid has been absorbed. Stir lemon juice in gently, taking care not to mash the beans. Transfer to a serving bowl and serve hot or at room temperature. Makes 4-5 servings.

Simmered Tofu and Vegetables

Savory baked tofu simmered in a delicate broth is not only the ultimate comfort food, but nourishes us deeply with the kinds of perfectly balanced nutrients that keep our bones strong and dense. And with miso in the broth, we'll digest more efficiently than we could ever imagine.

miso broth:
3 cups spring or filtered water
3-inch piece kombu

2 shallots, diced
1 carrot, diced
1 cup diced winter squash
1 cup small cauliflower florets
1 tablespoon barley miso
2 stalks broccoli, small florets
extra virgin olive oil
1 package flavored baked tofu
1-2 fresh scallions, thinly sliced on the diagonal

Place water and vegetables (except broccoli and scallions) in a medium soup pot over medium heat. Cover and bring to a boil. Reduce heat to low and cook until squash is tender, about 15 minutes. Remove a small amount of broth and puree miso. Stir miso back into broth with broccoli. Simmer 5-6 minutes, until the broccoli is crisp tender. Take care not to boil the miso as this will destroy the enzymes.

While the vegetables simmer, heat a small amount of oil in a skillet and quickly pan-fry the baked tofu, browning the edges, about 2 minutes per side.

To serve, spoon vegetables and broth into 4 individual bowls and top each one with a slice of baked tofu. Sprinkle with scallions and serve immediately. Makes 4 servings.

Fried Tofu on Steamed Bok Choy with Spicy Mustard Sauce

Now this is a main course! Feeding tofu skeptics? Try this dish on them . . . richly-flavored, light and fresh, this will satisfy even the fussiest eaters. And the nutrients? You have protein, calcium, vitamin C, magnesium, potassium and folic acid . . . and did I mention that it's delicious?

fried tofu:
4 tablespoons extra virgin olive oil
2 tablespoons brown rice syrup
1 tablespoon soy sauce
4 ounces extra firm tofu cut into 4 equal slices
4 baby bok choy, halved, rinsed very well

mustard sauce:
2 tablespoons extra virgin olive oil
generous pinch crushed red pepper flakes
4 tablespoons stoneground mustard
2 teaspoons brown rice syrup
2 teaspoons soy sauce
½ cup spring or filtered water
juice of ½ lemon

Place oil, rice syrup and soy sauce in a deep skillet over medium heat. Lay the tofu slices in the rice syrup mixture and reduce heat slightly. Fry the tofu until the edges have browned, 7-10 minutes.

While the tofu cooks, place bok choy in a bamboo steamer over boiling water. Cover and steam until bright green and crisp, about 4 minutes.

Make the sauce by combining all ingredients, except water and lemon juice in a sauce pan over medium heat. Bring to a boil and reduce heat to low. Slowly whisk in water to create a smooth, thick sauce. Remove from heat and whisk in lemon juice.

To serve, arrange bok choy on a serving platter with tofu slices on top. Spoon sauce over the dish and serve. Note that you may have more dressing than you need, so just serve it on the side. Makes 4 servings.

Fried Tempeh Sticks with Spicy Dipping Sauce

Tempeh and frying go together like love and marriage . . . just perfectly. And it's more than just taste that is so enchanting . . . with fat as the vehicle for eased digestion, you can rest assured of getting all the nutrients your precious bones need.

6 tablespoons extra virgin olive oil
2 tablespoons soy sauce
2 tablespoons brown rice syrup
8 ounces tempeh, sliced into thick strips
1 small bunch watercress, blanched, cut into bite-size pieces

dipping sauce:
½ cup spring or filtered water
½ small dried chili, finely minced
2 teaspoons soy sauce
½ teaspoon brown rice syrup juice of ¼ fresh lemon

Place oil, soy sauce and rice syrup in a deep skillet over medium heat. Just when the mixture begins to sizzle, lay the tempeh strips in, cover and reduce heat to low. Cook until browned, about 4 minutes. Carefully turn the tempeh strips and brown on the other side. Arrange watercress on a serving platter and lay tempeh strips on top.

Make the dipping sauce by combining all ingredients in a small sauce pan over low heat and cooking for 3-4 minutes, just to develop the flavors.

To serve, place the dipping sauce in a small bowl and serve with the fried tempeh and watercress. Makes 4-5 servings.

Lentil Curry

Ya' gotta love curry . . . and with lentils, it's pure heaven. The earthy spiciness blends so wonderfully with the oil, sautéed veggies and beans in this simple side dish. And what a delicious way to get our bones the nutrients they need.

Extra virgin olive oil
2-3 cloves fresh garlic, finely minced
½ red onion, diced
sea salt
½ teaspoon curry powder
½ red bell pepper, diced
½ yellow bell pepper, diced
1 cup baby green lentils, rinsed very well
2 ½ cups spring or filtered water
1 bay leaf
2-3 sprigs cilantro, finely minced

Place about 3 tablespoons oil, garlic and onion in a deep skillet over medium heat. When the onions begin to sizzle add a pinch of salt and curry powder and sauté for 1-2 minutes. Stir in peppers, a pinch of salt and sauté for 1-2 minutes. Stir in lentils and add water and bay leaf. Cover and bring to a boil. Reduce heat to low and cook until lentils are tender, about 45 minutes to one hour. When the beans are about 80% done, season to taste with salt and continue cooking until all liquid has been absorbed. Remove from heat and stir in cilantro. Serve hot or at room temperature with papadam. Makes 4-5 servings.

Black-Eyed Pea Fritters with Spicy Salsa

Black-eyed peas get a bad rap . . . everyone thinks of them as part of southern cuisine, humble beans of the poor . . . nothing more. Well, we could not be more wrong. These beans are powerhouses of nutrition essential to our bones . . . and we've brought them uptown in this richly flavored recipe with spicy salsa.

fritters:
extra virgin olive oil
1-2 cloves fresh garlic, finely minced
½ yellow onion, finely diced
sea salt
½ cup fresh/frozen corn kernels
1 cup cooked black-eyed peas
½ cup whole wheat pastry flour
½ cup semolina flour
light olive oil or avocado oil, for frying

spicy salsa:
¼ red onion, finely diced
½ fresh jalapeno, finely diced (do not seed)
2 vine-ripened tomatoes, diced (do not seed or peel)
5-6 oil-cured black olives, pitted, finely minced
½-2/3 teaspoon sea salt
2 teaspoons red wine vinegar
¼ cup extra virgin olive oil
3-4 sprigs fresh parsley, finely minced

Place about 2 tablespoons oil, garlic and onion in a deep skillet over medium heat. When the onion begins to sizzle, add a pinch of salt and sauté for 1-2 minutes. Stir in corn kernels and a pinch of salt and sauté for 1 minute. Stir in black-eyed peas, cover and cook over low heat for 3-4 minutes to develop flavors. Transfer to a mixing bowl and set aside to cool to room temperature. Mix in both flours and sea salt to taste, mixing to form a stiff batter. Form the batter into 2-inch round or oblong disks that are about ½-inch thick.

Place about ¼ inch light olive or avocado oil in a deep skillet and place over medium heat. When patterns form in the oil, called 'dancing,' the oil is hot enough to fry the fritters.

Preheat the oven to 275o. Fry fritters a few at a time, transfer to a parchment paper-lined baking sheet and place fritters in warm oven while frying the remainder.

Prepare the salsa by simply mixing together all the ingredients, adjusting seasoning to your taste. To serve, simply arrange fritters on a platter with salsa on the side. Makes about 12 servings.

Dandelion Greens with Cannellini Beans and Avocado

Bitter greens and beans are a classic Mediterranean combination that is not only delicious, but ensures that our precious bones get all the nutrients they need by supporting the function of the liver. And add to it the essential fatty acids that are some of the wonders of avocados and hempseeds and you have perfection.

Extra virgin olive oil
2-3 cloves fresh garlic, thinly sliced
1 red onion, thin half moon slices
sea salt
generous pinch crushed red pepper flakes
1 cup dried cannellini beans, rinsed very well
2 ½ cups spring or filtered water
½ cup dry white wine
1 bay leaf
1 small bunch dandelion, rinsed very well
grated zest of 1 lemon
2 ripe avocados, halved, pitted and thinly sliced
¼ cup shelled hempseeds, lightly pan toasted*

Place about 3 tablespoons oil, garlic and onion in a deep skillet over medium heat. When the onions begin to sizzle, add a pinch of salt and the red pepper flakes and sauté for 2-3 minutes. Add cannellini beans, water, wine and bay leaf and bring to a boil. Reduce heat to low and cook until the beans are tender, about 50 minutes. Season to taste with salt. Coarsely chop the dandelion greens and stir into the bean mixture with lemon zest and cook, stirring frequently, for 5 minutes more.

To serve, arrange avocado slices on a platter and mound beans and greens in the center. Sprinkle with hempseeds. Serve hot. Makes 4-5 servings.

Note: To toast hempseeds, simply heat a dry skillet over medium-low heat and stir in seeds. Cook, stirring constantly until the seeds are fragrant. Transfer to a glass bowl and cool completely.

Chickpea Tabouleh with Hempseeds

Grains and beans are a classic combination of nutrients for human health. Every cuisine has put these two together to ensure the perfect balance of nutrition. And to up the ante just a little, we've added essential fatty acid-rich hempseeds to make sure we're well nourished on every level.

2 cups spring or filtered water
1 ¼ cups bulgur (cracked wheat)
1 medium bunch fresh parsley, finely minced
¼ cup chopped fresh mint
¼ cup shelled hempseeds
1 ripe tomato, diced, do not peel or seed
½ cup cooked chickpeas
2-3 fresh scallions, minced
1 small cucumber, diced, do not peel or seed
juice of 1 fresh lemon
3 tablespoons extra virgin olive oil
2 tablespoons hempseed oil
sea salt
1/3 cup coarsely chopped, pitted, oil-cured black olives

Bring water to a boil and stir in bulgur. Cover and turn off heat. Allow to stand, undisturbed, until all the liquid has been absorbed into the grain, about 15-20 minutes. Fluff bulgur with a fork and transfer to a mixing bowl. Mix in the balance of ingredients, salting to taste. Adjust seasonings to your desire. Cover and chill completely before serving. Makes 3-4 servings.

Miso Braised Tofu with Garlic Sautéed Kale

I know what you're thinking . . . here come the tofu recipes. Tofu is a rich source of protein, good quality fat and the other essential nutrients for which soy has been prized for generations in Asia. And when the recipe is as delicious as this one?

4 tablespoons extra virgin olive oil
3 tablespoons Suzanne's Specialties Maple Rice Nectar
2 tablespoons soy sauce
1 brick extra firm tofu, sliced into 1/3-inch thick slabs
extra virgin olive oil
3-4 cloves fresh garlic, finely minced

½ red onion, thin half moon slices
sea salt
generous pinch crushed red pepper flakes
1 small bunch kale, rinsed very well

Place oil, rice nectar and soy sauce in a skillet over medium heat. When the mixture begins to sizzle, carefully arrange tofu slices in the pan. Cook until browned and then turn and brown on the other side, (about 3 minutes per side).

While the tofu cooks, place a small amount of oil, garlic and onion in a skillet over medium heat. When the onion begins to sizzle, add salt and crushed red pepper flakes and sauté for 1-2 minutes. Coarsely chop the kale and stir into the skillet. Season to taste with salt and sauté until bright green and just wilted, about 2 minutes.

To serve, arrange kale on a serving platter with tofu slices on top. Makes 4-5 servings.

Fried Tofu with Broccoli, Ginger and Garlic

Fried tofu is a wonderful thing . . . mild-mannered tofu takes on a rich, smooth, sensual texture with flavor to spare. In this simple main course, we take protein-rich tofu and pair it off with the calcium and vitamins C and D so abundant in broccoli.

Light olive or avocado oil
1 brick extra firm tofu, cut into 1-inch cubes
Extra virgin olive oil
2-3 cloves fresh garlic, finely minced
5-6 thin slices fresh ginger, cut into very fine matchsticks
1 red onion, thin half moon slices
sea salt
generous pinch crushed red pepper flakes
1 small carrot, fine matchstick pieces
4-5 dried shiitake mushrooms, soaked until tender, thinly sliced
2-3 stalks broccoli, small florets
juice of 1 fresh orange
1 teaspoon arrowroot

Place about 3 inches of oil in a deep pot over medium heat. When the oil is hot (you will see patterns forming in the bottom of the pan, known as 'dancing'), raise the heat to high and fry the tofu, a few cubes at a time, until crisp and golden, drain on paper and repeat until all the tofu is fried.

Place a small amount of oil, garlic, ginger and onion in a wok or skillet over medium heat. When the onion begins to sizzle, add a pinch of salt, crushed red pepper flakes and sauté for 2-3 minutes. Add carrot, a pinch of salt and sauté for 1 minute. Add shiitake, a pinch of salt and sauté for 2 minutes. Stir in broccoli, season to taste with salt, cover and reduce heat to low, cooking until broccoli is bright green and crisp. Dissolve arrowroot in orange juice and pour into skillet, stirring constantly until a thin, clear glaze forms. Fold in fried tofu and stir gently to coat. Serve immediately. Makes 4-5 servings.

Fried Stuffed Tofu with Curried Vegetables

Tofu has a mild character, not much flavor, but packed with nutrients, making it the perfect backdrop for any flavors you desire. In this richly-flavored side dish, tofu provides the wrapping, so to speak, for spicy sautéed veggies, a delicious way to nourish our bones.

1 brick extra firm tofu, cut into 8 triangles
light olive or avocado oil, for frying

broth:
3 cups spring or filtered water
2 tablespoons soy sauce
1 bay leaf
extra virgin olive oil
½ teaspoon red curry paste
2-3 cloves fresh garlic, finely minced
½ red onion, finely diced
sea salt
1 small carrot, finely diced
1 stalk celery, finely diced
2-3 scallions, finely diced

Cut the tofu into 4 thick triangles. Cut each triangle in half, making them half the their original thickness.

Place about 3 inches of oil in a deep pot over medium heat. Heat the oil through; you will know it's hot enough when patterns, known as 'dancing' form in the oil. Fry the tofu until golden, drain on paper and set aside.

Combine ingredients for broth in a deep pot over medium heat. Place fired tofu triangles in broth, reduce heat to low and cook, uncovered, for 15 minutes. Drain well, discard broth and cool tofu to room temperature.

Heat about 2 tablespoons oil and curry paste in a skillet, stirring the paste into the oil until it becomes creamy. Stir in garlic, onion and a pinch of salt and sauté for 1-2 minutes. Add carrot, a pinch of salt and sauté for 1-2 minutes. Stir in celery, scallion and salt to taste and sauté for 3-4 minutes. Remove from heat and cool slightly.

Carefully pull open the slits in the tofu triangles. Using a small spoon, stuff sautéed vegetables into each pocket, filling abundantly. Arrange on a platter, each triangle standing on its end, displaying the stuffing. Serve hot. Makes 4-8 servings.

Braised Tempeh with Sweet Sesame Sauce

Tempeh is an Indonesian product made by fermenting whole soybeans, creating a strong flavor and a 'meaty' texture. And being fermented, its many nutrients are easy to digest. In this recipe, we braise it to crisp perfection and smother it in a calcium-rich sesame sauce.

4 tablespoons extra virgin olive oil
2 tablespoons soy sauce
2 tablespoons brown rice syrup
8 ounces tempeh, cut into 1-inch triangles
extra virgin olive oil
2-3 cloves fresh garlic, finely minced
1 red onion, thin half moon slices
sea salt
4 tablespoons sesame tahini
½-2/3 cup plain soymilk
2 tablespoons brown rice syrup
juice of ½ fresh lemon
3-4 sprigs fresh parsley, finely minced

Pan braise the tempeh by heating oil, soy sauce and rice syrup together in a skillet over medium heat. When the mixture begins to sizzle, lay tempeh triangles in the skillet and braise until lightly browned. Turn tempeh and brown other side. Set aside.

Place about 2 tablespoons oil, garlic and onion in a deep skillet over medium heat. When the onions begin to sizzle, add a pinch of sea salt and sauté for 2-3 minutes, until the onions are quite limp. Add sesame tahini and ½ cup soymilk, stirring constantly to create a creamy texture. Stir in rice syrup and salt to taste, stirring constantly, slowly adding more soymilk as needed to create a thick, smooth sauce. Remove from heat, stir in tempeh, lemon juice and parsley. Serve hot over brown rice or with noodles. Makes 3-4 servings.

Breakfast Scramble

Being active, with running and the gym regular parts of our lives, Robert and I sometimes need a little protein boost for energy first thing in the morning. And since eggs and bacon are just not an option . . . we'll pass on the saturated fats, thanks . . . this tofu-based scramble has become a regular on our breakfast table.

Extra virgin olive oil
1 yellow onion, thin half moon slices
sea salt
3-4 button or crimini mushrooms, brushed free of dirt, thinly sliced
1-2 stalks celery, thinly sliced on the diagonal
1 carrot, fine matchstick pieces
½ cup fresh/frozen corn kernels
1 brick extra firm tofu, coarsely crumbled
1-2 fresh scallions, finely diced

Place 2-3 tablespoons oil and onion in a deep skillet over medium heat. When the onions begin to sizzle, add a pinch of salt and sauté the onions for 2-3 minutes. Add mushrooms, a pinch of salt and sauté for 1-2 minutes. Stir in celery and carrot, a pinch of salt and sauté for 1 minute. Stir in corn, a pinch of salt and sauté for 1 minute. Finally, stir in crumbled tofu, season to taste with salt and cook, stirring for 2-3 minutes. Fold in scallion and transfer to a serving platter. Serve with lightly cooked greens and whole grain toast. Makes 3-4 servings.

Tempeh with Carrots, Lotus Root and Sauerkraut

Simple dishes are often the most delightful. In this main course, simple vegetables support the strong flavor of tempeh to create a centerpiece that is so delicious, no one will believe it was so simple.

Extra virgin olive oil
2 tablespoons soy sauce
8 ounces tempeh, cut into1-inch cubes
2-3 cloves fresh garlic, finely minced

2-3 slices fresh ginger, finely minced
soy sauce
generous pinch crushed red pepper flakes
1 red onion, thin half moon slices
1 carrot, fine matchstick pieces
6-8 thin slices fresh lotus root, half moons
grated zest of 1 lemon
3 tablespoons sauerkraut, drained well
juice of ½ fresh lemon
2-3 sprigs fresh parsley, coarsely chopped

Place enough oil in a deep skillet to generously cover the bottom with the soy sauce over medium heat. When the oil is hot, pan fry the tempeh until golden, turning once to ensure even browning. Set aside. Clean out the skillet.

Place about 2 tablespoons oil, garlic, ginger and onion in the same skillet over medium heat. When the onion begins to sizzle, add a dash of soy sauce and crushed red pepper flakes and sauté for 1-2 minutes. Stir in carrot, a dash of soy sauce and sauté for 1 minute. Stir in lotus root, lemon zest, a dash of soy sauce and sauté for 1 minute. Spread vegetables evenly over skillet and top with tempeh and sauerkraut. Cover, reduce heat to low and braise over low heat until vegetables are tender, about 10 minutes. Remove from heat and gently stir in lemon juice. Serve immediately, garnished with parsley. Makes 3-4 servings.

Tempeh Reuben Sandwich with Caramelized Onions

Man, oh, man, these are the most delicious sandwiches. Hearty, richly flavored, smothered in sweetly caramelized onions and melted soy cheese. Serve these babies with a fresh, crisp salad for a yummy and nutritious lunch.

Extra virgin olive oil
2 red onions, thin half moon slices
sea salt
dry white wine
extra virgin olive oil
8 ounces tempeh, halved crosswise and each half split to half its thickness
4 slices vegan soy cheese
8 slices whole grain bread
stoneground mustard
1 fresh tomato, thickly sliced
romaine lettuce leaves

Place a small amount of oil in a deep skillet over medium heat. Begin to sauté onions with a pinch of salt. Add a small amount of wine and continue to stir until onions begin to wilt. Reduce heat to low and continue cooking, stirring frequently until onions begin to reduce dramatically and turn a rich brown color. This can take as long as 40 minutes.

When the onions are about 80% done, place a generous amount of oil in a skillet over medium heat. Pan fry the tempeh on both sides browning evenly. Lay a slice of soy cheese on each piece of tempeh and allow to melt.

To assemble the sandwiches, spread mustard on 4 slices and lay tomato and lettuce on top. Lay tempeh and cheese on top of that, mound onions over the sandwich and the remaining bread on top. Makes 4 sandwiches.

Chapter 10

Fabulous Fish

Oh, boy . . . fish. This was a tough decision for me to make. Choosing to live as a vegan (and no, I don't preach or spray paint meat eaters . . .), I had some serious reflecting to do when Robert faced his bone crisis. He's a distance runner and needed the kind of protein that only some form of animal food could give him. He also needed the essential fatty acids available in fish. But knowing what I did about animal food, I couldn't very well feed him meat, the very type of food that would continue to rob his already fragile bones of desperately needed nutrients.

I had to set my personal choices aside and decide what was best for my husband's health. Research showed me that the protein in fish would serve his needs without depleting him. Good. But then I faced the crisis of conscience of farm-raised fish and those consequences . . . both environmentally and personally. More research showed me that farm-raised fish lacked many of the nutrients so essential to Robert's recovery, so the choice was easy . . . wild fish or no fish. Luckily, I have access to a fish monger who can get me the freshest natural fish available.

I still choose not to eat fish or animal food of any kind . . . and that works for me. Many people, however, particularly those people struggling with bone loss or trying to regain what they have lost, will very likely need the protein and accompanying nutrients that are present in natural wild fish. To those people, I say enjoy the fish you eat with gratitude to Mother Nature for all that she provides.

Basil Oil-Marinated Sole with Lemony-Daikon Salad

Fish is a great source of animal protein for those of us who feel that we need it. In this recipe, mild-mannered sole is enhanced by the brilliant sparkle of fresh basil . . . and to help you digest it easily . . . a slightly spicy daikon salad.

3, 6-ounce sole filets, rinsed well

basil oil:
¼ cup extra virgin olive oil
2 cloves fresh garlic, thinly sliced
8-10 fresh basil leaves
sea salt
½ cup dry white wine

lemony-daikon salad:
1 cup fine matchstick daikon
½ fresh lemon, very thin half moon slices
½ teaspoon sea salt
juice of ½ fresh lemon
3 sprigs fresh basil
3 lemon wedges

Combine oil, garlic, basil and a generous pinch of salt in a small saucepan over low heat. Cook for 4-5 minutes to infuse the oil with basil and garlic flavors. Remove from heat and cool to room temperature.

Marinate the fish by arranging them in a shallow dish. Pour basil oil and wine over the filets and sprinkle lightly with salt. Marinate for 15-30 minutes.

While the fish marinates, prepare the salad. Combine daikon and lemon in a bowl with salt and lemon juice. Rub the vegetables between your fingers and set aside to marinate for 15 minutes.

To cook the fish, transfer filets to a skillet and pour marinade over top. Cover and cook over medium-low heat until the fish is opaque. Carefully transfer fish to a serving platter. Cook remaining marinade over medium heat until it reduces and thickens slightly, about 5 minutes. Spoon marinade over fish.

Gently squeeze any liquid from the daikon and lemon and serve on the side of the fish. Serve immediately. Makes 3 servings.

Monkfish Tempura with Spicy Dipping Sauce

Oh, man . . . tempura style fish is so rich, so delicious, so satisfying . . . and the winning combo of protein and fat really nourish our bones.

tempura batter:
1 cup whole wheat pastry flour
½ cup semolina flour
generous pinch sea salt
generous pinch chili powder
1 teaspoon baking powder
1 tablespoon kuzu
1 bottle dark beer
light olive or avocado oil
12 ounces monkfish, cut into 1 ½-inch pieces

dipping sauce:
2/3 cup spring or filtered water
2 tablespoons soy sauce
1 teaspoon hot chili olive oil
1 scallion, finely minced
1 clove fresh garlic, finely minced
1 bunch watercress, lightly blanched, coarsely chopped

Prepare the tempura batter by mixing together flours, salt, chili powder and baking powder. Dissolve kuzu in a small amount of beer and stir into flour mixture. Slowly add beer, stirring constantly, until a thin batter forms, much like pancake batter. Set aside for 10 minutes.

Wash fish well and cut into pieces. Heat about 3 inches oil in a deep pot, over medium heat. When the oil is hot (you will know because patterns will form in the oil, called 'dancing'), dip the fish pieces in the batter and fry a few at a time, until golden and crispy.

To make the dipping sauce, combine the ingredients in a saucepan and warm over low heat for 3-4 minutes, to activate the 'heat' in the chili oil.

To serve, arrange watercress on a platter with tempura fish on top with dipping sauce on the side and serve immediately. Makes about 4 servings.

Grilled Salmon with Spicy Asparagus

Salmon is a heartier fish, so I love to serve it with a lighter vegetable side dish to balance all the flavors, textures and energies of the ingredients . . . with just a touch of spice to add some zip.

marinade:
½ cup dry white wine
3 tablespoons hempseed oil
1 tablespoon extra virgin olive oil

2 shallots, finely minced
2 cloves fresh garlic, finely minced
1/3 teaspoon sea salt
grated zest of 1 lemon
4, 4-6-ounce salmon filets

asparagus:
extra virgin olive oil
½ red onion, thin half moon slices
sea salt
generous pinch crushed red pepper flakes
1 bunch asparagus, tips snapped

Whisk together all marinade ingredients. Arrange filets in a shallow baking dish and spoon marinade over top. Marinate for 10-15 minutes.

To cook the salmon, heat a grill to medium. Carefully transfer salmon to a platter, reserving marinade. Place salmon filets on the hot grill, brushing frequently with marinade. Cook, turning once, until salmon is opaque.

While the salmon grills, place about 2 tablespoons oil and red onion in a skillet over medium heat. When the onion begins to sizzle, add a pinch of salt and red pepper flakes and sauté for 2-3 minutes. Lay asparagus on top, sprinkle lightly with salt and cook over low heat until asparagus is bright green and crisp-tender, about 4 minutes.

To serve, arrange salmon on a serving platter, with asparagus and onions arranged on top. Serve immediately. Makes 4 servings.

Pan Fried Tilapia with Spicy Lentil Salad

Fried fish and spicy beans are a combination that is richly flavored and nutrient-dense, just what our bones need to stay strong . . . or regain their strength, for that matter.

lentil salad:
1/2 cup baby green lentils, rinsed very well
2 cups spring or filtered water
1 bay leaf
extra virgin olive oil
2-3 cloves fresh garlic, finely minced
½ red onion, finely diced
sea salt
½ jalapeno pepper, finely minced, do not seed
1 vine-ripened tomato, finely diced, do not seed or peel

1-2 sprigs fresh basil, finely minced
fried tilapia:
½ cup yellow cornmeal,
generous pinch sea salt
generous pinch cracked black pepper
extra virgin olive oil
4, 4-6-ounce tilapia filets, rinsed very well
4 lemon wedges

Place lentils, water and bay leaf in a small pot over medium heat and bring to a boil, uncovered. Cover, reduce heat to low and cook until lentils are just tender, about 45 minutes. Drain off any remaining liquid.

Place about 2 tablespoons oil, garlic and onion in a deep skillet over medium heat. When the onion begins to sizzle, add a pinch of salt and jalapeno and sauté for 2-3 minutes. Stir in cooked lentils, season to taste with salt, cover and reduce heat to very low. Simmer for 4-5 minutes to develop the flavors. Stir in tomato and basil and remove from heat.

While the beans simmer, whisk the cornmeal and seasonings together. Place enough oil in a skillet to generously cover the bottom over medium heat. Dredge each filet in the cornmeal mixture and fry until golden and crisp. Turn the filets and fry until the other side is golden and crisp. Drain on paper.

To serve, arrange fried fish on a platter, with lentils mounded in the center and lemon wedges on the side. Serve immediately. Makes about 4 servings.

Poached Salmon with Fennel

Salmon is pretty hearty, as fish goes. A meaty texture, strong taste and incredibly dense nutrient profile almost demand a lighter cooking technique to create balance. In this dish, a simple poaching in white wine creates a gentle flavor, but don't worry, sautéed fennel steps up to the plate to keep things interesting for our palate . . . and to help digest the dense protein of the fish.

poached salmon:
4, 4-6 ounce salmon filets, rinsed very well
dry white wine
extra virgin olive oil
sea salt
cracked black pepper

sautéed fennel:
extra virgin olive oil
1 red onion, thin half moon slices

sea salt
2 teaspoons honey or brown rice syrup
1 small bulb fennel, very thinly sliced, leaves removed, 2 tablespoons reserved
juice of ½ lemon

To poach the salmon, arrange filets in a deep skillet. Add about 4 tablespoons oil, white wine to half cover the fish and a light sprinkle of salt and pepper. Cover and turn heat to medium. When the wine begins to boil, reduce heat to low and cook until salmon is opaque.

While the salmon cooks, place about 2 tablespoons oil and onion in a skillet over medium heat. When the onion begins to sizzle, add a pinch of salt and sauté for 2-3 minutes. Stir in honey and fennel, season to taste with salt and sauté until fennel just wilts, about 4 minutes. Remove from heat and stir in lemon juice.

To serve, arrange salmon on a serving platter with sautéed fennel over top. Sprinkle with reserved fennel leaves and serve immediately. Makes about 4 servings.

Green Tea-Marinated Salmon and Sautéed Vegetables

Want to nourish your bones? And the rest of you? This is the dish for you! Not only do we have the nutrients of salmon, protein, essential fatty acids, vitamins and minerals, but we marinate it in anti-oxidant-rich green tea to pack a nutritional punch . . . and to lighten things up a bit? Some sautéed veggies . . .

marinade:
¼ cup extra virgin olive oil
½ cup dry white wine
2 teaspoons green tea powder*
sea salt
4, 4-6-ounce salmon filets, rinsed very well

vegetables:
extra virgin olive oil
1 red onion, thin half moon slices
sea salt
generous pinch crushed red pepper flakes
1-2 stalks celery, thinly sliced on the diagonal
1 carrot, very fine matchstick pieces
1 yellow summer squash, very fine matchstick pieces
5-6 leaves escarole, rinsed very well
4 lemon wedges

Make the marinade by whisking together oil, wine, green tea and a generous sprinkle of salt. Arrange salmon in a shallow dish and pour marinade over top. Set aside to marinate for 10-15 minutes. Carefully transfer salmon to a deep skillet, pour marinade over top and turn heat to medium. Cover and bring to a boil. Reduce heat to very low and cook until the salmon is opaque.

While the salmon cooks, sauté the vegetables. Place about 2 tablespoons oil and red onion in a skillet over medium heat. When the onion begins to sizzle, add a pinch of salt and red pepper flakes and sauté for 1-2 minutes. Add celery, a pinch of salt and sauté for 1 minute. Add carrot, a pinch of salt and sauté for 2 minutes. Add yellow squash, a pinch of salt and sauté for 1 minute. Slice the escarole leaves into thin ribbons and stir into vegetables, season to taste with salt and sauté just until escarole wilts.

To serve, arrange salmon on a serving platter, mound vegetables on top, with lemon wedges on the side. Serve immediately. Makes about 4 servings.

The best choice for this is to purchase green tea complex capsules and open them to release the powder.

Slow-Roasted Halibut with Miso Sauce

When the weather is chilly, we need to hang on to every bit of heat we can. In this recipe we combine roasted halibut with braised sweet root vegetables and a miso sauce designed to keep us warm and help us digest the hearty protein of the fish.

miso sauce:
4 teaspoons mellow white miso
2 tablespoons light sesame oil
2 tablespoons hempseed oil
2 teaspoons honey or brown rice syrup
grated zest of 1 lemon
4, 4-6-ounce halibut filets
extra virgin olive oil
honey or brown rice syrup
sea salt
1 sweet potato, cut into 1-inch chunks
1-2 carrots, cut into 1-inch irregular chunks
1 red onion, cut into 8 wedges
5-6 cloves fresh garlic, peeled, left whole
4 lemon wedges
4 tablespoons pan toasted shelled hempseeds

Prepare the miso sauce by simply whisking ingredients together to create a smooth consistency. You may need to add a little water to thin the sauce, but add only by tablespoons, so that you don't thin the sauce too much.

Preheat oven to 325o. Arrange halibut in a shallow baking dish. Pour about ¼-inch water into the dish. Spread or spoon miso sauce over each filet, covering the top surface completely. Cover dish and bake until fish is opaque, about 25 minutes. Remove cover and return to oven to brown the top slightly.

While the fish cooks, place about 4 tablespoons oil, 2 tablespoons honey and a generous pinch of salt in a deep skillet over medium heat. Arrange vegetables in the mixture, avoiding overlap. Cover and turn heat to medium. When you hear sizzling, reduce heat to low, shake the pan gently to coat the veggies and cook until they are tender and browned, about 25 minutes.

To serve, arrange halibut on a platter with braised vegetables around the rim, sprinkle with hempseeds and serve lemon wedges on the side. Serve immediately. Makes about 4 servings.

Note: To pan toast hempseeds, heat a stainless steel skillet over medium-low heat. Cook hempseeds, stirring constantly, until lightly browned and fragrant. Transfer to a heat-resistant bowl and set aside.

Smoked Salmon and Avocado Rolls

We're talking so-o-o-o-o-o-o-o incredibly rich, with creamy avocado, strongly flavored smoked salmon all nestled in brown rice and wrapped in mineral-rich nori. It doesn't get better than this starter course.

3 sheets toasted sushi nori
2 cups cooked short grain brown rice
1 large piece smoked salmon, sliced into ribbons
2 avocado, halved, stone removed, thinly sliced
juice of 1 lemon

dipping sauce:
½ cup spring or filtered water
2 teaspoons soy sauce
generous pinch crushed red pepper flakes, ground
1 teaspoon brown rice vinegar

Lay a bamboo sushi mat or kitchen towel on a dry, flat work surface. Lay a sheet of nori, shiny side down, on the mat. With wet hands, press one-third of the rice firmly on the nori, about ¼-inch thick, covering the nori end to end, but leaving about an inch exposed on the edges closet to and furthest from you. Lay a few smoked salmon strips on the rice closest to you, with avocado strips on top. The salmon and avocado should lay, in strips, end to end on the rice. Squeeze some lemon juice over the avocado. Using the mat or towel as a guide, roll the nori around the rice, jelly-roll style, creating a firm cylinder. Using we fingers, seal the nori to the roll. Set aside and repeat with remaining ingredients to create 3 nori rolls.

Using a wet knife, slice each nori roll into 8 equal pieces and arrange them, cut side up, on a platter. Make the dipping sauce by simply whisking together ingredients, adjusting seasoning to your taste. Serve dipping sauce on the side of the nori rolls. Makes 5-6 servings.

Warm Monkfish with Olive Oil Poached Tomatoes, Green Beans, Black Olives

Monkfish is known as poor man's lobster because of its rich, buttery flesh and delicious flavor. In this dish, we bring lots of strong flavors together to create a rich, seductive, satisfying main course that brings nutrients to your bones as deliciously as anything I can imagine.

2 tablespoons extra virgin olive oil
2/3 cup dry white wine
sea salt
cracked black pepper
12 ounces monkfish, cut into 2-inch pieces

tomatoes:
5 tablespoons extra virgin olive oil
½ teaspoon chili paste
sea salt
4 plum tomatoes, halved, do not seed or peel
2 cups green beans, tips removed, left whole
1 red bell pepper, roasted over an open flame, peeled, seeded, sliced into thin
    ribbons
12-15 oil-cured black olives, pitted, left whole

Place oil, wine, a generous pinch of salt and pepper in a deep skillet over medium heat. Arrange monkfish in the skillet, cover and bring to a boil. Reduce heat to low and cook until fish is opaque.

While the fish cooks, place oil, chili paste and 2 generous pinches of salt in a skillet over medium heat. Cook, stirring, until the paste is thoroughly mixed into the oil. Lay tomatoes, cut side down in the oil and cook, uncovered, until they just begin to wilt, about 15 minutes.

While the fish and tomatoes cook, bring a pot of water to a boil and cook green beans until crisp and bright green, about 4 minutes. Drain and transfer to a mixing bowl. Mix in cooked monkfish, red pepper and olives and drizzle with olive oil.

To serve, mound monkfish and green bean mixture in the center of a serving platter with tomatoes, arranged cut-side up around the rim. Serve immediately. Makes 4-6 servings.

Wok-Sautéed Salmon with Sweet and Sour Fennel and Kumquats

Salmon is a hearty and lovely fish, with strong taste nutrition to spare. In this main course, it is combined with fennel, sautéed with a delicate sweet and sour sauce and for a little zip, some kumquats, whose delightfully sour taste bursts on your tongue with each and every bite.

extra virgin olive oil
2-3 cloves fresh garlic, thinly sliced
1 red onion, thin half moon slices
sea salt
1 carrot, fine matchstick pieces
1 small fennel bulb, leaves removed, bulb thinly sliced
2 tablespoons honey or brown rice syrup
grated zest of 1 lemon
½ cup dry white wine
4, 4-6-ounce salmon filets, rinsed very well
10-12 kumquats, rinsed very well
juice of 1 lemon

Place about 4 tablespoons oil, garlic and onion in a wok over medium heat. When the onions begin to sizzle, add a pinch of salt and stir-fry for 1-2 minutes. Add carrots, a pinch of salt and stir-fry for 1-2 minutes. Add fennel, a pinch of salt and sauté for 1-2 minutes. Stir in honey, white wine, salt to taste and lemon zest. Lay salmon filets on top, sprinkle lightly with salt, cover wok and reduce heat to low. Cook until fish is opaque. Remove cover and carefully transfer salmon to a serving platter. Stir kumquats into vegetables until just incorporated. Remove from heat and stir in lemon juice.

To serve mound vegetables and kumquats on top of salmon and serve immediately. Makes 4-6 servings.

Small Fried Fish with Fresh Lemon

When smelt is in season, in the late fall, my husband never misses a chance to batter and fry them up. He says they are heaven on a plate. Being vegetarian, this depth of emotion is lost on me, but I have mastered the way his mother cooked it . . . because nothing is better than a husband in culinary heaven.

batter:
1 cup whole wheat pastry flour
½ cup semolina flour
generous pinch sea salt
generous pinch chili powder
1 teaspoon baking powder
1 tablespoon kuzu
1 bottle dark beer
light olive or avocado oil
6-8 smelts, rinsed very well
8 lemon wedges

Make the batter by whisking together the flours and seasonings. Dissolve kuzu in a small amount of the beer and mix into flour. Slowly add beer to, while mixing, to create a thin, smooth batter, as you would for pancakes. Set aside for 15 minutes before proceeding.

To pan fry the fish, place about an inch of oil in a deep skillet over medium heat. When the oil is hot (you will know the oil is hot when patterns known as 'dancing' form in the oil), dip smelts in batter and fry until golden and crispy, turning once to ensure even browning. Drain on paper and repeat until all smelts are fried. Serve immediately with lemon wedges. Makes about 4 servings.

Sardine Spread

Sardines are another of my husband's favorites . . . and with good reason. One of the finest ways to get the nutrients we need to keep our bones healthy, sardines can be some of your bones' best pals. An acquired taste, this spread gentles their strong flavor, making a rich and delicious sandwich spread.

1 can sardines in oil or water
3-4 scallions, finely minced
2-3 cloves fresh garlic, finely minced
½ red onion, finely minced

3 tablespoons stoneground mustard
1/3 cup non-dairy mayonnaise
sea salt
cracked black pepper
scant pinch chili powder
juice of ½ lemon

Place sardines in a small mixing bowl and coarsely mash them with a fork. Stir in balance of ingredients, mixing well with the fork. Adjust seasonings to your taste. Chill completely before serving.

To serve, spread thickly on whole grain bread with lettuce and tomato. Makes about 2 sandwiches.

Baked Stuffed Monkfish

The rich flavor and buttery texture of monkfish makes it a total delight to eat. In this recipe, stuffed with a slightly spicy breadcrumb filling, humble monkfish shines as a main course fit for a king . . . and his bones!

stuffing:
extra virgin olive oil
1-2 cloves fresh garlic, finely minced
½ red onion, finely diced
sea salt
generous pinch crushed red pepper flakes
1 stalk celery, finely diced
1 small carrot, finely diced
dry white wine
1 cup whole wheat bread crumbs
1-2 sprigs fresh basil, leaves removed, finely minced
12 ounces monkfish, rinsed well

Preheat oven to 375o.

Place about 2 tablespoons oil, garlic and onion in a deep skillet over medium heat. When the onion begins to sizzle, add a pinch of salt, crushed red pepper flakes and sauté for 2-3 minutes. Stir in celery, a pinch of salt and sauté for 1 minute. Stir in carrot, a pinch of salt and sauté for 1 minute. Add about ½ cup white wine, season to taste with salt and cook, stirring, until liquid is absorbed into veggies. Stir in breadcrumbs and basil and remove from heat.

Wash fish and lay in a shallow baking dish. Using sharp knife, make a slit along the top of the fish, creating a deep crevice for the filling. Spoon breadcrumb mixture into crevice, filling abundantly. Drizzle with olive oil. Pour white wine into baking dish to accumulate about ½ inch in the bottom of the dish. Cover tightly and bake until fish is opaque, about 25 minutes. Remove cover and continue baking until topping is lightly browned. Makes 3-4 servings.

Steamed Tilapia with Lemon Sauce

Light and fresh-tasting, tilapia is a wonderful way to add the nutrients of fish to your diet. In this dish, the delicate taste and flaky texture of this white fish is showcased with a simple, zesty lemon sauce.

2-3 leaves Chinese cabbage, rinsed well, leaves left whole
2 lemons, thinly sliced
4, 4-6 ounce tilapia filets, rinsed well
sea salt
cracked black pepper
extra virgin olive oil

lemon sauce:
¼ cup spring or filtered water
½ cup dry white wine
sea salt
½ teaspoon kuzu, dissolved in small amount cold water
juice of 1 fresh lemon
2-3 sprigs fresh parsley, finely minced

Arrange cabbage leaves over the surface of a bamboo steamer with lemon slices on top. Arrange the filets on the lemon slices, season lightly with salt and pepper and drizzle with olive oil. Cover and set steamer over a deep skillet of boiling water. Cook until fish is opaque.

While the fish cooks, place water, wine and a generous pinch of salt in a small sauce pan over low heat. When the mixture has heated through, stir in dissolved kuzu and cook, while stirring until the mixture thickens slightly. Remove from heat and whisk in lemon juice, creating a smooth sauce.

To serve, arrange fish filets on a platter, spoon sauce over top. Lay some lemon slices from the steamer on top of the fish and sprinkle with parsley. Serve immediately. Makes about 4 servings.

Haddock en Papillotte

Simple and yummy . . . some of the most important culinary jargon I know. This dish has it all . . . richly flavored fish and lots of tender, succulent vegetables . . . all coming together to nourish our precious bones.

4, 12-inch x 12-inch pieces parchment paper
1 red onion, thin half moon slices
1 carrot, fine matchstick pieces
1 cup fine matchstick daikon
1 cup finely shredded green cabbage
1 red bell pepper, roasted over an open flame, peeled, seeded, sliced into thin
    ribbons
extra virgin olive oil
sea salt
balsamic vinegar
4, 4-6-ounce haddock filets, rinsed well

Preheat oven to 350o. Lay parchment paper on a dry work surface.

Place cut veggies in a mixing bowl and drizzle generously with oil, sprinkle with salt and stir in a sprinkle of balsamic vinegar. Toss to coat.

Lay a haddock filet on each piece of parchment, sprinkle lightly with salt and drizzle with oil. Mound equal portions of veggies on each filet. Wrap parchment, sandwich style around the fish and veggies (lift up 2 sides, roll them to the center of the fish, fold the other sides into points and wrap under fish). Arrange packets in a shallow baking dish, avoiding overlap and bake for 25 minutes. Open one packet and check to see if fish is opaque. If so, remove from oven, open packets and transfer fish and vegetables to a serving platter. Serve immediately, garnished with lemon wedges. Makes 4-5 servings.

Chapter 11

Vitalizing Vegetables

How much time do you have to listen to me wax on about the importance of vegetables in our daily diet? I could rant for days about their value and how diets lacking them are leading to our demise . . . and it ain't a pretty demise, either. Stooped over spines, fragile hips, aching, brittle, immobile joints are all the direct result of not enough vegetables in our diets. Think I'm kidding? Sure, the key to healthy bones is balanced eating with nutrients from all sorts of foods, but I have to tell you . . . vegetables are the kings, queens, princes, dukes and duchesses of nutrition.

Walking into a supermarket tells us all we need to know about health. What's the first section of the market to greet you? Fresh produce, abundantly stacked and artfully arranged. How many times have you wandered through displays of fruits and vegetables, struck by the beauty and vitality surrounding you, overcome with the freshness, the color, the perfumes of the food? Why do you suppose that happens?

The word 'vegetable' comes from the Latin verb meaning 'to enliven.' A beautiful produce display strikes with vibrant colors, but what *really* attracts you to is the sheer magnetism of life in its freshest, purest state. You identify with the living energy. I would venture to guess that impulse buying is less compelling in the canned vegetable aisle. To be surrounded by fresh, living vegetables makes us feel alive and vital.

Fresh vegetables are enlivened by the combination of the energies of the sun, earth, water and air, creating a balanced vitality essential for life. Without vegetables in our diet, we grow weak. Disconnected from nature's life-giving energy, we find ourselves lost, searching for ways to strengthen and enliven ourselves. We take supplements, energy drinks, vitality bars; we ingest pills, take shots and concoct potions on the quest for energy and vitality—and eternal youth and beauty. And it ain't there, because life ain't there. Vegetables give us so much life. Vegetables, as the original source of protein on earth, give us protein in its purest form. Think about it . . . you can eat vegetables and go directly to the source of the strength—avoiding the middle cow or pig or chicken. Vegetables are the greatest source of vitamins and minerals on the planet. From folic acid to vitamin C, D and many members of the B family to useable calcium to any other nutrient you can imagine, you'll find them, in abundance, in vegetables. But as important as the fiber and vitamins and protein and carbohydrates are to our health and our bones, I am much more enchanted by the incredible energy we get from glorious vegetables.

Look at root vegetables. They drill into the soil, drawing nutrients into their deep roots. They are firmly lodged in the ground; they know exactly where they are going—no waffling here. Including them in our diet brings similar energy into the body. Eating root vegetables—carrots, parsnips, turnips, rutabaga, daikon, burdock—makes us stronger. Root vegetables root us to the ground, keep us focused and clear. Drilling into the soil as they grow, they draw nutrients deep into the body, so that we feel deeply nourished when we eat them. The intestines, in turn, have the job of influencing the quality of blood that nourishes the organs that, in turn, nourish our cells and our bones.

And the there are the round, sweet vegetables that grow close to the ground . . . winter squash, head cabbage, onions, Brussels sprouts, to name a few. With their calm, quiet natures and delicious sweet flavors, these are the vegetables that help you keep your cool; help you stay calm and serene. These are the perfect de-stress foods. Relaxing the middle organs, particularly the spleen and pancreas helps the body to release toxins effectively and to regulate our blood sugar, preventing stagnant energy and erratic emotions, which can result in tense, tight muscles and stiff bones as we struggle to cope with the ups and downs of our turbulent lives.

Ah, the leafy greens. In my humble opinion, these simple vegetables, kale, collard greens, watercress, mustard greens, bok choy, broccoli rabe, dandelion, arugula, are some of the most important foods we can consume to put our best face forward. Rich in anti-oxidants, calcium, vitamins C and D, iron, magnesium and folic acid, these leaves may look delicate, but they are incredible sources of strength. Drawing nutrients completely into their leaves from their delicate roots means that the leaves are thoroughly nourished. Their rich green color is indicative of rich sources of chlorophyll, which through photosynthesis will oxygenate our blood, improving the strength of our hemoglobin (red blood cells). And that means strong, dense bones.

And then there is the energy of the greens, with their cooling and adaptable natures. Greens will grow in any weather—hot, dry, wet or cold, snow, rain or drought—indicating that they are quite adaptable. That energy will be reflected in us, giving us a relaxed, flexible nature, relaxed, flexible muscles and bones that are not brittle. With greens, life's little adventures won't leave us looking drawn and exhausted. We develop an ability to roll with the punches, remaining flexible, but strong . . . no pushovers, these greens. Survival in any weather may indicate an adaptable nature, but also strength.

Exotic sea plants are more than just unique. Rich in protein, calcium, vitamins and minerals that enrich our organs, blood and bones, these strong vegetables are essential to maintaining strong, well-balanced vitality. Small amounts of these dense nutrients insure that we nourish our organs with essential nutrients for health.

The vitality of life and beauty that we all crave so deeply is within easy grasp—in the humble bins of any farmers' market, natural food store or supermarket. They can be found in broccoli, carrots, onions, kale and simple green cabbage, to name but a few gems in the crown of nature. To take your nutrients from the food you eat, instead of from pills, drinks or other supplements (except where absolutely necessary), brings more to your body than vitamin C, folic acid and iron. You get to ingest the nutrients, of course, but more importantly, you merge with the energy of nature—the sun, the earth, the water, the air. You re-connect with nature, nourishing yourself the way we nourish our beautiful plants and flowers, with energy and vitality—and life.

Avocado, Corn and Pepper Salad

Essential fatty acids are vital to bone health, particularly omega-3. Without it, we can become deficient and lose bone density. In this richly flavored salad, we get precious omega-3 from both avocado and hempseeds, nourishing our bones deliciously.

2 cups baby arugula, rinsed very well, left whole
2 ripe avocados, halved, seed removed, thinly sliced
2 ears fresh corn, kernels removed
2 red bell peppers, roasted over an open flame, peeled, seeded, sliced into thin ribbons

dressing:
3 tablespoons extra virgin olive oil
1 tablespoon hempseed oil
1 teaspoon raw honey
juice of ½ fresh lemon
sea salt
cracked black pepper
¼ red onion, finely minced
2 cloves fresh garlic, finely minced

2 sprigs fresh basil, finely minced
1-2 tablespoons shelled hempseeds, lightly pan toasted

Arrange arugula on a platter. Fan avocado slices around the rim. Mix together corn and peppers and mound in the center of the platter.

Make the dressing by whisking together oils, honey and lemon juice. Season to taste with salt and pepper and whisk well. Stir in onion, garlic and basil.

To serve, simply spoon dressing over the salad and sprinkle hempseeds on top. Serve immediately. Makes 2-3 servings.

Guacamole with Corn and Chile

A twist on traditional guacamole . . . a little corn, whose sweetly flavored carbohydrate energy will lighten up the density of the dish and a little spice to help digest the valuable nutrients in this delicious dip.

2 ripe avocados, halved, seeds removed, flesh removed from skin
1 tablespoons extra virgin olive oil
sea salt
generous pinch chili powder
juice of ½ fresh lemon
1 vine-ripened tomato, diced
½ cup fresh/frozen corn kernels
½ red onion, finely minced
1-2 cloves fresh garlic, finely minced
1-2 sprigs fresh cilantro, finely minced

Place the avocado flesh in a mixing bowl and mash with a fork to create a smooth paste. Stir in oil, salt to taste, chili and lemon juice, mixing until smooth. Stir in tomato, corn, onion, garlic and cilantro. Adjust seasonings to your taste. Cover and chill completely. Serve with tortilla chips or vegetable sticks. Makes 3-4 servings.

Squash Blossoms Stuffed with Avocado, Corn and Peppers

In the spring and the autumn, one of Mother Nature's wonders is squash blossoms . . . the beautiful, succulent flowers atop fresh zucchini. Thinly sliced in salads, sautéed, stirred into risotto or stuffed, as in this recipe . . . they are stunning.

4 zucchini blossoms, left whole, stamen removed
extra virgin olive oil
1 cloves fresh garlic, finely minced
¼ red onion, finely diced
sea salt
scant pinch crushed red pepper flakes
1 stalk celery, finely diced
½ carrot, finely diced
¼ cup fresh/frozen corn kernels
1 avocado, halved, seed removed, mashed

Clean the blossoms and remove the stamens without opening the flowers too much.

Place about 2 tablespoons oil, garlic and onion in a skillet over medium heat. When the onions begin to sizzle, add a pinch of salt and crushed red pepper flakes and sauté for 1-2 minutes. Stir in celery, a pinch of salt and sauté for 1 minute. Stir in carrot, a pinch of salt and sauté for 1 minute. Stir in corn, a pinch of salt and sauté for 1-2 minutes. Season lightly with salt and sauté until the veggies are crisp-tender, about 4 minutes. Remove from heat, transfer to a mixing bowl and cool to room temperature. Stir in avocado until ingredients are well-incorporated.

Using a spoon, stuff the blossoms abundantly. Set aside. Place enough oil in a deep skillet to accumulate ¼-inch over medium heat. When the oil is hot (you'll know the oil is hot when patterns form in the oil, known as 'dancing'), pan fry the blossoms until the flowers are crisp and golden, turning frequently to ensure even browning.

Drain well and serve fried blossoms on a bed of fresh salad greens. Makes 2-4 servings.

Black Bean, Pumpkin Seed and Chile Salsa

I love salsa . . . and when you know how nutrient-packed the ingredients are in salsa, you'll settle down to that heaping bowl of salsa with chips on the side with a whole new attitude and love it, too. From protein and trace minerals to lycopene and essential fatty acids, what a delicious way to nourish our bones.

1 cup cooked black turtle beans, half mashed
extra virgin olive oil
2-3 cloves fresh garlic, finely minced
½ red onion, finely minced

sea salt
½ fresh jalapeno pepper, finely minced (do not seed)
1-2 vine-ripened tomatoes, diced, (do not seed or peel)
grated zest of 1 fresh lemon
juice of ½ fresh lemon
½ cup pumpkin seeds, lightly pan toasted
1-2 sprigs fresh cilantro, finely minced

Place beans in a mixing bowl and mash with a fork until they are half broken.

Place about 2 tablespoons oil, garlic and onion in a skillet. When the onions begin to sizzle, add a pinch of salt and sauté for 1 minute. Stir in jalapeno, a pinch of salt and sauté for 1 minute (to release the heat). Remove from heat, transfer to a mixing bowl and cool to room temperature.

When the vegetables are cooled, stir them into the mashed beans with the balance of ingredients, except pumpkin seeds and sea salt to your taste. Chill completely so the flavor develops. Just before serving, stir in pumpkin seeds and serve with organic corn chips. Makes 3-4 servings.

Tomato Salad with Corn and Slivered Almonds

Rich in lycopene, vitamin C, magnesium and folic acid, tomatoes are a great addition to a healthy diet. And don't worry about the acid and your bones. By cooking, marinating or drying tomatoes, the acid is neutralized and you get to enjoy all the yummy nutrients this lovely, succulent fruit offers . . . and we added almonds for a touch of protein and essential fatty acids.

extra virgin olive oil
½-1 teaspoon chili paste
1-2 cloves fresh garlic, thinly sliced
1 red onion, thin half moon slices
sea salt
4 vine-ripened tomatoes, halved lengthwise, do not peel or seed
1 cup fresh/frozen corn kernels
2-3 sprigs fresh basil, leaves removed, leaves left whole
2 cups baby arugula, rinsed well, left whole
½ cup slivered almonds, lightly pan toasted
fresh lemon juice

Place about 2 tablespoons oil and chili paste in a skillet over medium heat. When the oil heats up, stir until the chili paste and oil turns creamy. Stir in garlic, onion and a pinch of sea salt and sauté for 1-2 minutes. Spread onions and garlic evenly over the bottom of the skillet and lay tomatoes, cut side down on the onions. Cover, reduce heat to low and cook just until tomatoes wilt, 7-10 minutes. Add corn and basil, season to taste with salt, do not stir. Cook for 3 minutes. Arrange arugula on a serving platter. Using tongs, carefully lift tomato halves from skillet and arrange them, cut side up on the arugula. Stir the corn and basil into the onions. Spoon the onion mixture over the tomatoes and sprinkle with almonds. Finish with a drizzle of olive oil and fresh lemon juice, if desired. Makes 4-5 servings.

Veggie Ragout of Artichokes, Greens and Chickpeas

Ragout is the most amazing, cozy and warming food . . . richly-flavored, satisfying and comforting . . . not to mention nutrition-packed. Use any variety of hearty, cold weather vegetables and beans to create your own masterpiece of a main course!

extra virgin olive oil
2-3 cloves fresh garlic, thinly sliced
2 red onions, thick wedges
sea salt
2 tablespoons honey
generous pinch crushed red pepper flakes
scant pinch cinnamon
grated zest of 1 lemon
1 carrot, 1-inch irregular cut chunks
1 parsnip, 1-inch irregular chunks
2 globe artichokes, trimmed, cut into quarters
1 cup cooked chickpeas
1 cup dry white wine
1 small bunch broccoli rabe, rinsed well, finely cut

Preheat oven to 325o.
    Using a deep pot that can move from stovetop to oven, place it over medium heat. Spoon 3-4 tablespoons oil in the pot with garlic and onions. When the onions begin to sizzle, add a pinch of salt, honey, crushed red pepper flakes, cinnamon, lemon zest and sauté for 2-3 minutes. Stir in carrots and parsnips, a pinch of salt and sauté for 2 minutes. Arrange vegetables evenly on the bottom of the pot and lay artichokes on top, with chickpeas on top of the artichokes. Add wine and sprinkle lightly with salt. Cover tightly and bake for 25-30 minutes. Remove cover, return to oven and bake until any remaining liquid has reduced and been absorbed into the dish. Remove from oven and stir in finely cut broccoli rabe until it wilts. Serve immediately. Makes 4-5 servings.

Oven-Roasted Winter Squash with Curried Hempseeds

Sweet, satisfying, nourishing, delicious and so nutrient-packed. It doesn't get better as a side dish than this simple, richly flavored baked winter squash.

3 cups 1-inch cubes of winter squash
extra virgin olive oil
sea salt
maple-flavored brown rice syrup
grated zest of 1 fresh lemon
curried hempseeds:
1 teaspoon curry powder
pinch sea salt
6 tablespoons shelled hempseeds

Preheat oven to 375o.

Place squash cubes in a mixing bowl. Drizzle generously with oil, sprinkle lightly with salt, drizzle with rice syrup and add lemon zest. Stir well to coat squash. Transfer to a shallow baking dish, avoiding overlap. Cover tightly and bake for 45 minutes. Remove cover and return to oven and brown the edges of the vegetables.

While the squash cooks, place a stainless steel skillet over medium heat. Dry roast curry powder for 3 minutes. Stir in hempseeds and cook, stirring constantly until the seeds are fragrant, about 3 minutes. Remove from heat and transfer to a heat-resistant bowl and cool completely. You will have more curried hempseeds than you will need, so once cooled, transfer the condiment to a glass jar that seals. It will keep for about 4 weeks.

To serve, simply sprinkle lightly with curried hempseeds and serve hot. Makes 4-5 servings.

Braised Carrots and Brussels Sprouts with Hempseed Vinaigrette

Braised vegetables are so delicious and so easy to make . . . there is no excuse for not eating well . . . and yummy? Give this a try . . . and see for yourself. And did I mention that it's nutrient-packed as well?

extra virgin olive oil
½ cup dry white wine
2-3 cloves fresh garlic, split in half lengthwise
1 red onion, diced

sea salt
2 cups baby carrots
12-15 Brussels sprouts, stems trimmed

hempseed vinaigrette:
3 tablespoons extra virgin olive oil
1 tablespoon hempseed oil
sea salt
cracked black pepper
1 shallot, finely minced
grated zest of 1 fresh lemon
juice of 1 lemon
1 teaspoon shelled hempseeds, lightly pan toasted
4-8 lemon wedges

Place about 2 tablespoons oil, wine, garlic, red onion and a generous pinch of salt in a deep skillet. When the onions begin to sizzle, add baby carrots, Brussels sprouts and a light sprinkling of salt, cover and reduce heat to low. Cook until vegetables are tender and beginning to brown, about 25 minutes. Remove cover and cook off any remaining liquid.

While the vegetables cook, simply whisk together oils, salt and pepper to taste, shallot, lemon zest and juice until a smooth, emulsified dressing forms. Stir in hempseeds.

To serve, toss vegetables gently with dressing, transfer to a serving platter and serve with lemon wedges on the side. Makes 4-5 servings.

Burdock Kinpira

The Japanese call this dish 'golden pieces.' I call it 'rocket fuel.' It's so jam-packed with nutrients, so richly flavored, so strengthening, so perfectly balanced, it's no wonder that legend says it takes us to enlightenment.

extra virgin olive oil
4-5 slices fresh ginger, fine matchstick pieces
1 cup fine matchsticks burdock
sea salt
generous pinch crushed red pepper flakes
1 cup fine matchstick carrots
soy sauce
2-3 sprigs fresh parsley, finely minced

Place about 2 tablespoons oil in a cast iron skillet over medium heat. When the oil is hot, stir in ginger, burdock, a pinch of salt and red pepper flakes and sauté for 2 minutes. Stir in carrot, season lightly with soy sauce and sauté until veggies are tender, 4-5 minutes. Remove from heat and stir in parsley. Serve hot. Makes 3-4 servings.

Burdock Eel

This is one of those dishes that you have to experience to appreciate. It's a little bit of work, to be sure, but the end result is so rich, so delicious, so nutrient-packed, with just enough fat to carry all those nutrients to where they are needed . . . you won't want to miss this one.

tempura batter:
1 cup whole wheat pastry flour
½ cup semolina flour
pinch sea salt
1 teaspoon baking powder
2 teaspoons kuzu, dissolved in small amount cold water
1 bottle dark beer (or sparkling water)
light olive or avocado oil
2 medium/large burdock, sliced into thin diagonal pieces
2 yellow onions, thin rings

dashi:
2 cups spring or filtered water
2-3 tablespoons soy sauce
1-inch piece kombu
4-5 slices fresh ginger
2 dried shitake mushrooms, soaked until soft

Preheat oven to 325o.

Make the tempura batter by whisking together dry ingredients. Dissolve kuzu and stir into flour mixture. Slowly add beer, stirring constantly to create a thin batter, like that for pancakes. Cover loosely and set aside for 15 minutes.

Place about 3 inches oil in a deep pot over medium heat. When the oil is hot (you will know it's hot when you see patterns forming, known as 'dancing'), raise the heat to high. Working with a few pieces at a time, dip burdock and onion slices in batter and fry until golden brown. Drain on paper, and repeat until all the veggie pieces are fried.

While frying, make the dashi. Simply combine ingredients in a sauce pan and cook over medium-low heat for 7-10 minutes.

When all the veggies are fried, arrange them in a baking dish. Strain dashi, discarding vegetables from the broth. Slowly pour dashi over fried vegetables until they are generously covered. Cover baking dish tightly and bake for 2-3 hours, until the veggies have 'melted' into the dashi. Remove cover and return to oven to brown for 5 minutes. Serve immediately. Makes 5-6 servings.

Composed Salad with Avocado

There is nothing as elegant as a composed salad plate . . . with vegetables arranged like a masterpiece. The combination here is not only artful and gorgeous, but contains balanced nutrition for our bones.

hempseed vinaigrette:
4 tablespoons extra virgin olive oil
1 tablespoon hempseed oil
2-3 teaspoons red wine vinegar or lemon juice
1-2 teaspoons raw honey
sea salt
cracked black pepper
1 tablespoon shelled hempseeds

salad:
3 cups baby arugula, rinsed well, left whole
12-16 oil-cured black olives, pitted, left whole
1 red bell pepper, roasted over an open flame, peeled, seeded, diced
2 vine-ripened tomatoes, diced, do not seed or peel
1 small cucumber, diced, do not seed or peel (only peel if not organic)
2-3 ripe avocados, halved, seed removed, thinly sliced

Make the vinaigrette by whisking together oils, vinegar and honey. Stir in salt and pepper to taste and hempseeds. Set aside so the flavors can develop while making the salad.

Arrange arugula on a platter. Combine olives, red pepper, tomatoes and cucumbers in a mixing bowl. Pour 2/3 of the dressing over the vegetables and toss to coat.

Mound dressed vegetables in the center of the arugula, with avocado slices arranged around the rim. Drizzle balance of dressing over avocado and arugula and serve immediately. Makes 4-5 servings.

Bitter Green Salad with Dulse Sprinkle

I always say that whenever you think you have eaten enough dark green vegetables, eat more. It's not really a joke. These humble veggies are jam-packed with nutrients for our bones from calcium and vitamin C to folic acid, magnesium and phosphorus. And delicious? Give them a try. And with the mineral punch of dulse in this salad, you really can't lose.

1 small bunch watercress, rinsed well, hand shredded
2 cups baby arugula, rinsed well
1 red or green Belgian endive
3-4 red radishes, halved, thinly sliced into half moons
1 small cucumber, diced (do not seed or peel)
1 small carrot, shredded
2 tablespoons extra virgin olive oil
1 tablespoon hempseed oil
sea salt
cracked black pepper
juice of ½ fresh lemon
1-2 teaspoons dulse flakes

Place all vegetables in a mixing bowl. Stir in oils, a light sprinkle of salt and pepper and lemon juice. Toss well to coat. Arrange salad on a platter or in a shallow bowl and sprinkle with dulse flakes. Serve chilled or at room temperature. Makes 3-4 servings.

Lemony Endive Salad

Bitter greens benefit our health in so many ways, from aiding in the digestion of fats and proteins to helping to cleanse and tonify our very overworked livers. In this simple and elegant salad, we combine bitter greens with a delightfully tart dressing to keep our energy sparkling.

3-4 Belgian endive, bottoms trimmed, leaves removed, left whole
1 red onion, very thin half moon slices
3 tablespoons extra virgin olive oil
sea salt
cracked black pepper
juice of 1 fresh lemon
1 teaspoon honey
6-8 oil-cured black olives, pitted

Place endive leaves and onion in a mixing bowl. Whisk together oil, a generous pinch of salt, black pepper to taste, lemon juice and honey until smooth. Pour over endive and toss to coat. Arrange dressed endive mixture on a serving platter with olives on top. Serve at room temperature or chilled. Makes 4-5 servings.

Garlic Sautéed Greens

What? More greens? I told you . . . you can never get enough! Jam packed with minerals, folic acid, vitamin C, biologically available calcium, chlorophyll, potassium and magnesium, dark leafy greens are the key to vitality and strong bones.

Extra virgin olive oil
4-5 cloves fresh garlic, thinly sliced
1 red onion, thin half moon slices
sea salt
generous pinch crushed red pepper flakes
1 small bunch kale, collard greens, broccoli rabe or other dark green, rinsed
     well, left whole
4 lemon wedges

Place about 3 tablespoons oil, garlic and onion in a skillet over medium heat. When the onions begin to sizzle, add a pinch of salt, the chili flakes and sauté for 1-2 minutes. Just before you are ready to sauté them, slice the greens into bite-sized pieces and add to skillet. Season to taste with salt and sauté until just wilted and a rich green color, about 3 minutes. Transfer to a serving platter and serve immediately with lemon wedges on the side. Makes 3-4 servings.

Braised Broccoli Rabe with Roasted Red Peppers and Hempseeds

This is a side dish that will have you and your loved ones in love with greens. Don't let the spicy zip and the rich flavor fool you. The nutrients in this simple side dish are just perfect for keeping your bones healthy . . . from calcium and folic acid to omega 3.

Extra virgin olive oil
2-3 cloves fresh garlic, finely minced
1 yellow onion, diced

sea salt
cracked black pepper
1 fresh jalapeno pepper, finely minced, with seeds
1 red bell pepper, roasted over an open flame, peeled, seeded, sliced into thin
    ribbons
1 small bunch broccoli rabe, rinsed well, stems trimmed, left whole
dry white wine
2 teaspoons shelled hempseeds, lightly pan toasted

Place about 3 tablespoons oil, garlic and onion in a deep skillet over medium heat. When the onions begin to sizzle, add a pinch of salt and pepper and sauté for 2-3 minutes. Stir in jalapeno and roasted peppers, a pinch of salt and sauté for 1-2 minutes. Stir in broccoli rabe, season lightly with salt and drizzle with wine. Cover, reduce heat to low and braise broccoli rabe until wilted and bright green, about 4 minutes. Stir well to combine ingredients and transfer to a serving platter. Sprinkle with hempseeds and serve immediately. Makes 3-4 servings.

Braised Turnips and Tops

Turnips are a great source of the nutrients our bones need, from calcium to folic acid to vitamin C and D. Richly braised, they are a side dish that you will savor . . . as will your bones.

4 tablespoons extra virgin olive oil
1 teaspoon sea salt
2 tablespoons balsamic vinegar
4 baby turnips with tops, rinsed very well, left whole

Place oil, salt and vinegar in a deep skillet and arrange turnips and tops in the liquid. Cover the place over medium-low heat. When you hear sizzling, gently shake the skillet to coat the turnips with the cooking liquid. Cook until turnips can be easily pierced with a fork, about 20 minutes. The greens will be quite wilted. Transfer turnips to a serving platter. Cook any remaining liquid in the skillet until a thick syrup forms. Spoon over turnips and serve immediately. Makes 2-3 servings.

Note: If you can not find baby turnips, use full sized turnips with tops. Split them, lengthwise, keeping greens attached and lay them, cut side down in the skillet to braise.

Curried Cabbage with Sesame Sauce

Simple humble green cabbage shines in this recipe, lightly curried with a creamy sesame glaze. But there's nothing humble about the power of cabbage in our day to day health. Prized for thousands of years for its anti-inflammatory and antibiotic prowess, this cooling, gentle vegetable will keep you calm and cool.

Extra virgin olive oil
1 teaspoon red curry paste
2-3 cloves fresh garlic, thinly sliced
1 yellow onion, thin half moon slices
sea salt
½ head green cabbage, cut into 1-inch chunks
3 tablespoons sesame tahini
juice of ½ fresh lemon
1 teaspoon brown rice syrup or honey
1-2 teaspoons black sesame seeds, lightly pan toasted

Place about 3 tablespoons oil and curry paste in a deep skillet over medium heat. Cook, while stirring, until the curry paste is incorporated into the oil. Stir in garlic and onion, a pinch of salt and sauté for 1-2 minutes. Lay cabbage chunks on top, season lightly with salt, cover and reduce heat to low. Cook until cabbage wilts, about 12 minutes.

For the sauce, whisk together tahini, salt to taste, lemon juice and sweetener with enough water to create a thick, smooth sauce.

Remove cabbage from heat and stir in sesame sauce to coat. Transfer to a serving platter and sprinkle with sesame seeds. Serve hot. Makes 3-4 servings.

Sautéed Escarole Salad

Another way to get dark leafy greens. This hot salad combines the brilliance of sautéing with crisp, fresh vegetables to create a delicious variety of taste and texture . . . anything to get you to eat greens!

Extra virgin olive oil
2-3 cloves fresh garlic, thinly sliced
1 red onion, thin half moon slices
sea salt

generous pinch crushed red pepper flakes
1 small head escarole, rinsed very well, leaves hand shredded
1 small cucumber, diced, do not seed or peel
1-2 vine ripened tomatoes, diced, do not seed or peel
2-3 sprigs fresh basil, leaves removed, left whole
juice of ½ fresh lemon

Place about 2 tablespoons oil, garlic and onion in a deep skillet over medium heat. When the onions begin to sizzle, add a pinch of salt, red pepper flakes and sauté for 1-2 minutes. Lay escarole on top, season lightly with salt, cover and reduce heat to low. Cook just until escarole wilts, 2-3 minutes. Remove from heat and stir in cucumber, tomatoes and basil. Transfer to a serving platter and drizzle with olive oil and lemon juice. Serve immediately. Makes 3-4 servings.

Hiziki Caviar on Daikon and Carrot Canapés

Sea plants, while exotic to many of us, are valuable foods for maintaining strong, healthy bones. Nutrient-rich, these little plants can be strong, so we only need a tiny amount for them to make a difference in our health. This elegant starter is a great way to add sea plants to your diet.

Extra virgin olive oil
3-4 cloves fresh garlic, finely minced
3-4 slices fresh ginger, finely minced
½ red onion, finely diced
2-3 shallots, finely minced
sea salt
½ cup dry hiziki, soaked until tender, finely minced
dry white wine
soy sauce
12-16 carrot rounds, steamed until crisp-tender
12-16 daikon rounds, steamed until crisp-tender
1-2 sprigs fresh parsley, finely minced

Place about 2 tablespoons oil, garlic, ginger, onion and shallots in a small skillet over medium heat. When the vegetables begin to sizzle, add a pinch of salt and sauté for 3-4 minutes. Spread vegetables over the bottom of the skillet and top with hiziki. Add enough white wine to half cover ingredients. Season to taste with soy sauce, cover, reduce heat to low and cook until hiziki is tender, about 30 minutes. Remove cover and continue cooking until any remaining liquid has reduced to a thin syrup. Stir well to combine.

To serve, lay a carrot round on top of each daikon round and mound hiziki on top. Arrange on a serving platter and sprinkle with parsley. Serve warm or at room temperature. Makes 4-6 servings.

Hiziki Turnovers

Richly flavored sea plants wrapped in tender, flaky pastry . . . who says healthy cooking can't taste yummy?

Light sesame oil
3-4 slices fresh ginger, finely minced
soy sauce
½ cup dried hiziki, soaked until tender, finely diced
mirin
½ cup fresh/frozen corn kernels
2-3 fresh scallions, finely diced

pastry:
1 cup whole wheat pastry flour
½ cup semolina flour
pinch sea salt
½ teaspoon baking powder
2-3 tablespoons light olive or avocado oil
spring or filtered water
2-3 teaspoons shelled hempseeds

Place oil in a small sauce pan over medium heat. When the oil is hot, sauté ginger, with a splash of soy sauce for 1 minute. Stir in hiziki, season to taste with soy sauce, add a generous sprinkle of mirin and enough water to half cover. Bring to a boil, cover, reduce heat to low and cook until hiziki is tender, about 25 minutes. Remove cover and cook away any remaining liquid. Stir in corn and scallions. Set aside to cool to room temperature.

Prepare the pastry by combining flours, salt and baking powder in a mixing bowl. Using a fork or pastry cutter, cut in oil to create the texture of wet sand. Slowly add water, while mixing to create a stiff, rollable dough. Gather into a ball, wrap in plastic and allow dough to rest until hiziki is cooled.

To assemble the turnovers, roll out dough into a rectangle, about 1/8-inch thick. Cut into 3-inch squares. Lay a square on a dry work surface. Spoon about 3 tablespoons hiziki onto the center of the square. Lift one corner of pastry, fold over filling and press onto the opposite corner, creating a triangular turnover. Using a wet fork, seal the edges of the turnover. Repeat with balance of ingredients.

Preheat oven to 350o and line a baking sheet with parchment. Arrange turnovers on baking sheet, brush with oil and sprinkle lightly with hempseeds. Bake until pastry is golden and firm to the touch, 25-30 minutes. Makes 4-5 servings.

Hiziki Strudel

Another richly flavored way to serve nutrient-packed hiziki. The richest of all sea plants in useable calcium, as well as other trace minerals, this is one sea plant you don't want to miss.

Extra virgin olive oil
1-2 cloves fresh garlic, finely minced
½ red onion, diced
sea salt
generous pinch crushed red pepper flakes
2/3 cup dried hiziki, soaked until tender, diced
soy sauce
dry white wine
1 carrot, diced
1 small zucchini, diced
1 small yellow squash, diced
3 sheets whole wheat phyllo dough*
1-2 tablespoons shelled hempseeds

Place about 2 tablespoons oil, garlic and onion in a deep skillet over medium heat. When the onions begin to sizzle, add a pinch of salt, red pepper flakes and sauté onion for 1-2 minutes. Spread onions evenly over skillet and top with hiziki. Season to taste with soy sauce and sprinkle generously with mirin. Add white wine to half cover ingredients, cover and bring to a boil. Reduce heat to low, add carrot, zucchini and yellow squash (but do not stir in) and cook until hiziki is tender, about 25 minutes. Remove cover and cook away an remaining liquid. Set aside to cool to room temperature before proceeding.

Lay a sheet of phyllo on a dry flat work surface. Brush with oil and sprinkle with hempseeds. Lay a second sheet on top, brush with oil and sprinkle with hempseeds. Lay the third sheet on top and brush with oil. Spoon cooled hiziki over phyllo, leaving 1 inch of phyllo exposed on the edge closest to you and on either side, covering as much of the phyllo as possible. From the narrow edge, closest to you, roll the phyllo around the filling, jelly-roll style, rolling and folding the edges in to seal the ends of the strudel.

Preheat oven to 350o and line a baking sheet with parchment. Lay the strudel on the lined baking sheet. Using a sharp knife, make deep slits in the strudel, to allow steam to escape and to mark servings. Brush lightly with oil and bake until the phyllo is lightly browned and crisp, about 20 minutes. Remove from oven and allow to cool for 10 minutes before slicing.

To serve, slice strudel and arrange, cut sides up on a serving plate. Serve warm or at room temperature. Makes about 8 servings.

Note: Purchase phyllo dough frozen and thaw in the refrigerator over several hours to ensure even thawing and no soggy parts.

Sesame Hiziki Salad

This richly flavored warm salad is laced through with veggies and smothered in a creamy sauce to create a side dish fit for a king . . . and great for your bones.

½ cup dried hiziki, soaked until tender, diced
soy sauce
mirin

salad:
extra virgin olive oil
1-2 cloves fresh garlic, finely minced
2-3 slices fresh ginger, finely minced
½ small leek, rinsed free of dirt, thinly sliced
1 carrot, fine matchstick pieces
2-3 red radishes, thinly sliced
½ small cucumber, very thin half moon slices
1 bunch watercress, rinsed well, sliced into bite-sized pieces

sesame dressing:
2-3 tablespoons sesame tahini
grated zest of 1 fresh lemon
juice of ½ fresh lemon
2 teaspoons honey
soy sauce

Place hiziki in a sauce pan, discarding soaking water. Add soy sauce to taste, a generous pinch of mirin and spring or filtered water to half cover the hiziki. Cover and bring to a boil. Reduce heat to low and cook until hiziki is tender, about 25 minutes. Remove cover and cook away any remaining liquid.

Place about 1 tablespoon oil, garlic, ginger and leek in a skillet over medium heat. When the leek begins to sizzle, add a splash of soy sauce and sauté for 1-2 minutes. Stir in carrot, a splash of soy sauce and sauté for 1-2 minutes more. Vegetables will still be crisp. Set aside to cool.

Arrange radishes, cucumber and watercress on a platter and chill completely.

Make the dressing by whisking tahini, lemon zest and juice, honey and a light sprinkle of soy sauce until smooth. Slowly whisk in water to create a smooth sauce.

Mix hiziki and sautéed veggies together with dressing and mound on the platter of watercress. Serve immediately. Makes about 4 servings.

Kombu Pickle

Pickled foods, like fermented foods are an important part of a healthy diet. They are one of the best ways to optimize digestion. To pickle a sea plant renders it very digestible, making the nutrients readily available to us . . . and our bones.

6, 3-inch strips of kombu, soaked until tender, sliced into 1-inch pieces
4 tablespoons umeboshi vinegar
juice of ½ fresh lemon
2 teaspoons honey

Lay kombu in a shallow bowl. Whisk balance of ingredients together and toss with kombu pieces. Cover with cheesecloth and set aside in a cool place (no the refrigerator), to pickle for 24-48 hours. When pickled to your taste, transfer to a small glass jar, liquid and all, and refrigerate.

You need only a couple of pieces of this pickle for a serving. Pickles will keep for up to 3 weeks. Makes 8-10 servings.

Nori Pesto

I learned this recipe from a great teacher, Shizuko Yamamoto, not only a brilliant shiatsu practitioner, but a fine, creative and rich cook. Simple nori comes to life with hot spicy flavors, nuts and oil to make a richly flavored, nutrient-rich . . . and yummy pesto.

Extra virgin olive oil
3-4 cloves fresh garlic, finely minced
½ red onion, finely diced

sea salt
1 jalapeno pepper, finely minced, seeds and all
3-4 sheets toasted sushi nori, finely shredded
½ cup walnut pieces, pine nuts or pumpkin seeds
4-5 sprigs basil, leaves removed
2 teaspoons honey

Place about 2 tablespoons oil, garlic and onion in a small skillet over medium heat. When the onions begin to sizzle, add a pinch of salt and sauté for 1-2 minutes. Stir in jalapeno, a pinch of salt and sauté for 2 minutes to release the heat. Stir in nori, season very lightly with salt, cover and cook over low heat until nori is soft and creamy, about 4 minutes.

Place nuts or seeds, basil and honey in a food processor and add nori mixture. Puree until smooth.

To serve, cook some noodles and spoon a small amount of pesto on top. Makes 3-4 servings.

Dulse Hempseed Sprinkle

Condiments are our way of balancing each dish we eat for our own personal tastes. In this strongly flavored version, we create a sprinkle rich in trace minerals, potassium, magnesium, iron from the dulse . . . and protein, omega-3 and amino acids from the hempseeds. Delicious and good for our bones . . . perfect.

¼ cup dried dulse, loosely packed
6 tablespoons shelled hempseeds

Place a stainless steel skillet over medium heat. Dry roast dulse until crisp and fragrant, about 3 minutes. Transfer to a mortar and pestle and grind dulse into a fine powder.

In the same skillet, dry roast hempseeds over low until fragrant, about 3 minutes. Take care not to burn the seeds.

Transfer seeds and dulse to a small bowl and stir to combine. Cool completely before transferring to a glass jar. This condiment will keep, in a sealed jar, for about 3 weeks. Use only ½ teaspoon per serving. Makes about 2/3 cup.

Chapter 12

Delicious Desserts

What do desserts have to do with healthy bones? A lot, if you are eating sweets laden with fat, simple sugars and all manner of chemicals. It may taste great, but is, quite literally, poison . . . and deadly for our bones. It doesn't have to be that way—you can have your cake and eat it, to coin a phrase.

The body responds most dramatically to sweet flavor. It satisfies, relaxes, centers; it makes us happy; it leaves us feeling sated and contented. Think about it. Ever find yourself absolutely craving another hearts of lettuce salad when you're stressed, upset, happy or looking to celebrate? We don't create birthday stews or wedding onion rings? We celebrate with sweet cakes.So what's the deal with dessert? Good for us or bad? It can be both, depending on what's in it. Desserts made with white flour, sugar, heavy cream, milk, eggs, colorings, flavorings and chemicals will, at the very least, make us fat and lethargic, with mood swings that can rival the highest roller coasters. On top of that, they don't really satisfy our taste for sweet—we think they do, but the reality is that these kinds of foods only make us want more of them. Why? Simple sugar and simple carbohydrates (white flour). These foods send your glycemic index into such a tailspin that the only way to stability is to load up on more sugar.

The real answer is to break the pattern of sugar highs and lows. And while that's not always easy, it's the only answer. The best news is that giving up simple sugar doesn't condemn you to a grim existence with no sweet treats in the picture. It's just a matter of switching around a few ingredients, making healthier choices. You will still create delicious, satisfying desserts, but you will create them with ingredients that leave you in charge of when you eat them, not the other way around. And wouldn't the world be a lovely place with you controlling your life, rather than your life being controlled by chocolate (which is decidedly different than loving chocolate and choosing it as a treat)?

As our world drives us harder and harder, with more and more pressure to perform—and to do it quickly, our bodies become more and more stressed, literally becoming rigid with tension, as our muscles tighten and our bones stiffen to protect us from the shocking reality that is our modern world. On top of that, we consume great quantities of animal protein, which makes the body hard and rigid externally and tired and stressed internally, as it struggles to assimilate the density of the food.

There are many ways in which we attempt to relax the body, most of them not very healthy. Drink, drugs, excessive eating, junk food, sugar can all be attempts to relax tension in the body. See if it's true for you. When you're feeling particularly tense after a day at the office, do you rush off to a yoga class for inner peace? Or do you fall into a chair with a bag of chocolate chip cookies and sink into a sugar-induced, mind-numbing stupor? In each case, you extract yourself from the circumstances that have created tension, but while the yoga (or other exercise) opens and relaxes the body and strengthens the bones, the sugary cookies simply numb you.

And simple, refined sugar's effect on our bones? Robbing us of vitamins, trace minerals and other nutrients essential to the health of our bones, sugar has been linked by several studies to loss of bone density. And since sugar makes you fat (no sugar-coating here) . . . you're a heavier weight on your fragile bones . . . are you connecting the dots here? However, if the desserts you are choosing are of superior quality, made from fresh, whole ingredients—whole grain flours and sweeteners, organic, seasonal fruit, nuts and other healthy items—then dessert takes on a whole new face, so to speak. Not only does it satisfy your sweet desires, but there's no compromise to your health in the process. Is it a bit more work to eat healthier treats, since you'll need to make most of them? Yes, of course. Are your bones worth the effort? It is, if you want to eat dessert and live to tell about it.

Kind of makes indulgence take on a whole new meaning, doesn't it?

What Goes Into Healthy Sweets

What goes into a healthy dessert? First, remember that dessert isn't medicine. It is to be enjoyed, not prescribed. While not an indulgence, dessert isn't a food group either. Dessert is designed to create an air of celebration, not to create more anxiety in our lives.

When it comes to dessert creation, I am unwilling to compromise on health, quality of ingredients and taste and appeal. So how do we create enjoyable, healthful desserts? How do we bake light, moist cakes and muffins; flaky pie crusts and pastries; rich, chewy cookies? How do we avoid creating those whole foods desserts that have the taste and texture of, well, healthy desserts?

My years of cooking naturally and creating all manner of recipes have taught me that the key is to make healthful desserts *seem* like indulgences. It is possible to balance the demands of healthy foods with the sensual pleasures of eating. We can eat well without giving up one of our most precious indulgences—dessert—and taste.

It is learning, through experimentation and practice, how the ingredients you are using will work together. Just bear in mind that the ingredients may change, but the techniques remain the same. For example, conventional cakes are light, moist and springy to the touch due to the companioning of eggs, white flour, milk and sugar, as well as intense whipping during the mixing process (imparting air into the batter for that familiar light texture). Whole-grain-based cakes will never yield exactly that texture. However, you *can* create a light, moist cake that has full-bodied taste and texture.Let's talk about some tips, techniques and of course, ingredients. I use only whole wheat pastry flour when baking cakes, cookies, pie crusts, pastries, muffins, tortes, cupcakes or other baked treats. It is a finer grind of flour, ground from a softer strain of wheat—quite different from regular whole wheat flour (which is great for breads, but not desserts)—and creates in a lighter end product. I very rarely use white flour—bleached or unbleached—in my baking. It is highly refined and compromised, nutritionally deficient and really tough on the digestive tract. However, sometimes I combine whole wheat pastry flour with semolina flour when essential to the final outcome. But that is rarely the case, especially when I can achieve satisfactory results without it.

Assemble all the ingredients you will need before you begin to bake. Preheat your oven and prepare your cake pans or sheet pans before you begin. This will allow you to work quickly. You want to mix the batter and bake it. You don't want it sitting for several minutes while you prepare your pans and heat your oven. Letting the batter sitting for several minutes will cause it to saturate itself, again, resulting in a heavy end product.

When mixing ingredients, use pastry knives, forks, spoons—anything but your hands. The oil from your skin will coat the flour and can create a tough, spongy dough. Handle the dough only when necessary, or as a recipe requires. Don't knead dough unless the recipe requires it; and when it does, don't over-knead—or under-knead. Inexperienced bakers would do well to follow recipes to the letter until certain techniques are mastered and you develop a "feel" for the doughs and batters.

Equally important is achieving satisfying flavor. Sweet doesn't mean heavenly. It takes more—depth of flavor is where dessert really soars. Conventional desserts have the benefit of lots of fat, dairy and artificial ingredients to impart rich taste. Healthful desserts must be a tad bit more creative to deliver satisfaction.

To create moist textures in your pastries, you need a fat or fat substitute. Conventional baked goods rely on milk, cream, eggs, butter, margarine or artificial fat additives. Since I choose not to cook with any of those foods, viable alternatives had to be discovered. My past experience has shown corn oil to be the clear winner, imparting a buttery flavor unsurpassed by other oils and creating a tender crumb and flavorful pastry. However, with the use of genetically modified corn in the pressing of corn oil, it became clear to me that it was no longer an option. I was looking through some old family recipes and found a pound cake that was made with light olive oil instead of butter. I had a culinary epiphany and began to scour old Italian cookbooks and found that light olive oil is used with great frequency in desserts. I worked through all the basics—pie crusts, cookies, pastry, cakes, even pancakes—and the results are so dreamy that I can't wait for you to give these recipes a try. Substitute olive oil in any recipe where you are using corn or canola (or whatever) for spectacular results. Citrus zest . . . adding citrus zest to a recipe is a sensational way to add depth of flavor to desserts. The zest is the colored part of the outer skin of lemons, oranges and other citrus fruits and adds a tangy zip to fruit compotes, sauces, cakes, pastries and puddings. Since zest only has a mild sweet zing to it, you can pretty much use it as you desire.

Eggs are used in desserts for two reasons—to leaven and/or to bind. There are a couple of alternatives to eggs in dessert-making. For leavening, you may simply add one teaspoon of non-aluminum baking powder for every egg in the recipe.

In recipes where eggs act as binders, I have simply substituted one teaspoon dissolved kuzu or arrowroot for each egg and have been quite successful. For custards or flan, a combination of agar flakes and kuzu have proved most satisfying in providing a firm, creamy pudding. Usually a teaspoon of each—kuzu and agar—is enough to yield the firmest, creamiest custards.

Which brings us to dairy substitutes. With the popularity of soymilk soaring, it should be no surprise to discover that it is a great milk substitute. Another option for milk, especially for custards and cream fillings, amasake, a sweet, fermented rice milk, is brilliant and delicately sweet. You may also choose from the many grain and nut milks available.

Nuts are a most wonderful addition to healthful desserts for many reasons. Their fat content give desserts a rich, distinctive flavor and their texture adds an interestingly appealing crunch. And they are a great source of plant protein.

Since sugar will kill us, literally, what's the alternative? The best quality sweeteners I have found are grain-based. Barley malt, brown rice syrup, wheat and oat malt are the sweeteners I choose. The beauty of grain sweeteners is that they are mostly complex sugars, not simple sugars, so they are released into the blood slowly, providing fuel for the body instead of creating ups and downs we experience when we eat simple sugars. They are simply whole grains, inoculated with a fermenting agent and then cooked until they reduce to a syrup.

Rice syrup yields a delicate sweetness that is very satisfying, with no aftertaste. It is the perfect sweetener for most cakes, pastries, cookies and puddings. Barley, wheat and oat malts have a stronger taste, much like molasses, so I reserve their use for desserts that complement that kind of taste, like spice cakes, carrot cakes, pumpkin pie and caramel sauces.

And then there's honey. Used for centuries to treat anemia and other weakening ailments, honey is rich in vitamins, minerals and antioxidants. It is also an inverted sugar, meaning that it doesn't ferment in the intestines and so doesn't affect blood chemistry as dramatically as other simple sugars. So, in small amounts, honey can be a great treat.

I rarely use maple syrup or fruit sweeteners, again, because they are simple sugars and also because they have such a strong sweet taste, which can overpower the other dessert flavors. Grain sweeteners yield a lovely sweet taste . . . just enough to be satisfying, but won't make our teeth hurt.

The most important thing to remember is that desserts should always taste like an indulgence . . . or they are not worth the work or the calories.

Marinated Nectarines and Berries

Fruit desserts are light and fresh . . . and just perfect after any meal. For ideal digestion, however, simply wait to eat dessert for about 20 minutes . . . which may be hard with a treat like this one!

2-3 ripe nectarines, halved, seeded, diced (do not peel)
½ cup ripe raspberries, rinsed well
½ cup ripe blueberries, rinsed well
½ cup ripe blackberries, rinsed well
pinch sea salt
juice of ½ fresh lemon
3-4 tablespoons honey

Place fruit in a mixing bowl. Toss gently with a pinch of salt. Whisk together lemon juice and honey. Gently toss fruit with honey mixture to coat the fruit. Chill completely before serving. Makes 3-4 servings.

Note: I like to serve this fruit salad garnished with toasted unsweetened coconut.

Lemony Pomegranates

When I was a kid, the only thing that made the passing of Christmas passable was, what we called, Chinese apples . . . but we now know as pomegranates. Totally delicious, delicately tart and slightly exotic, the jewel-like seeds of this fruit don't need very much enhancement . . . as you will see . . . oh, and the nutrients . . . off the charts with polyphenols, those splendid compounds that keep us strong and healthy.

2 pomegranates, split*, seeds removed
juice of ½ fresh lemon
2 teaspoons honey
pinch sea salt

Place pomegranate seeds in a small bowl and toss with remaining ingredients until coated. Chill completely before serving. Makes 3-4 servings.

Note: To open a pomegranate, make slits dividing the fruit into 4 equal sections. Place thumbs in the top and pull fruit open, revealing seeds.

Poached Pears in Plum Sauce

Light, fresh, low in the simple sugars that can rob our bones of nutrients, this dessert is as satisfying as one can get. Elegant, flavorful and substantial, without being heavy, this is a dessert to cap off any meal.

3 ripe, but still firm pears, peeled, left whole
spring or filtered water
2 cinnamon sticks
2 whole lemons, quartered
3 tablespoons brown rice syrup

plum sauce:
2 ripe plums, split lengthwise, stones removed, diced
4 tablespoons unsweetened raspberry jam
2 tablespoons brown rice syrup
grated zest of 1 lemon
pinch sea salt
scant pinch chili powder

Place the pears in a deep pot, standing on their ends. Pour in enough water to cover the pears by one third. Add cinnamon sticks, lemon wedges and rice syrup. Cover and bring to a boil. Reduce heat to low and cook pears until they can be easily pierced with a fork. Remove from cooking liquid and transfer to a plate.

While the pears cook, make the plum sauce. Combine all ingredients in a sauce pan and cook over medium-low heat until fruit is very soft, about 25 minutes. Transfer the sauce to a chinois, creating a smooth sauce.

To serve, spoon sauce on 3 individual dessert plates, reserving some sauce. Stand a pear in the pool of sauce on each plate. Spoon remaining sauce over pears. Garnish with fresh mint or fresh berries, when in season. Makes 3 servings.

Stewed Summer Fruit

We all love fresh summer fruit, crisp, juicy, lush . . . and that's just grand . . . but if you want a rich decadent-tasting . . . but totally without guilt treat, try stewing delicate summer fruit in a sweet sauce . . . satisfying, yummy and with no cost to the health of your bones.

2 ripe peaches, halved, stones removed, diced
2 ripe plums, halved, stones removed, diced
pinch sea salt
3 tablespoons honey
juice of ½ fresh lemon
6-8 strawberries, stems removed, quartered
½ cup raspberries, rinsed very well

Place peaches and plums in a sauce pan with salt and honey. Cook over low heat just until peaches are tender, about 4 minutes. Remove from heat, stir in lemon juice and berries. Spoon into individual serving cups and chill completely before serving. Makes 4-5 servings.

Poached Fresh Figs

There is not a more sensual fruit than a fresh fig. Lush, sweet, juicy . . . with soft flesh that yields to your every wish. They literally make you weak with their tender sweetness. But they're not just sexy . . . they are a fine source of many of the nutrients our precious bones need to stay strong. Lightly poached, as in this recipe, they're even easier to digest . . . sweet!

6-8 fresh figs, rinsed well
spring or filtered water
1 cinnamon stick
pinch sea salt
grated zest of 1 lemon
2 tablespoons honey
juice of ½ fresh lemon

Place figs in a sauce pan. Add water to half cover. Add balance of ingredients, cover and bring to a boil over medium heat. Cover and reduce heat to low. Cook figs just until tender, 7-10 minutes. Do not over cook. Transfer figs to a serving plate. Continue cooking liquid until it reduces to a thin syrup. Remove cinnamon stick and discard. Spoon reduced liquid over figs and sprinkle with lemon juice. Serve immediately. Makes 4-6 servings.

Fresh Berries in Champagne Sauce

Think there's nothing finer than fresh berries? This recipe may change your mind. You know the old seduction trick of eating strawberries with champagne to intensify the heady sweetness of the fruit? Nothing gets sexier than this dessert . . . or easier.

10-12 fresh strawberries, rinsed well, stems removed, halved

champagne sauce:
1 cup champagne pinch sea salt
2 tablespoons honey
grated zest of 1 orange
several sprigs fresh mint

Arrange strawberry halves on a plate and chill completely. Make the sauce while the berries chill. Combine champagne, salt, honey and orange zest in a small sauce pan and place over medium heat. Cook, uncovered, until the sauce reduces to a thick syrup.

To serve, spoon sauce onto 4 individual serving plates. Pile strawberries on top and serve garnished with mint leaves. Makes 4 servings.

Rice Pudding with Fresh Apricot Sauce

Creamy, delicately spiced . . . the ultimate comfort food . . . rice pudding. And to up the ante and increase nutrients for our bones, we top it off with a sweet and tart apricot sauce . . . yum!

pudding:
½ cup Arborio rice, do not rinse
3 cups vanilla soymilk
1 teaspoon pure vanilla extract
½ cup honey
pinch sea salt
scant pinch cinnamon
scant pinch ground ginger

apricot sauce:
4-5 fresh apricots, halved, pitted, diced
½ cup dry white wine
pinch sea salt
3 teaspoons honey
grated zest of 1 fresh lemon
2 tablespoons shelled hempseeds, lightly pan toasted

Place all rice pudding ingredients in a heavy pot over medium-low heat and bring to a boil. Cover and reduce heat to low and cook until rice is quite creamy and the liquid has become thick, stirring frequently, for as long a 1 ½ hours.

While the rice simmers, make the apricot sauce. Combine all ingredients, except hempseeds, in a sauce pan over medium-low heat. Cook, uncovered, until the apricots break down and the sauce gets creamy, about 20 minutes.

To serve, spoon rice pudding into individual dessert cups and spoon some apricot sauce on top. Serve warm or at room temperature. Makes 4-5 servings.

Stewed Dried Fruit

My husband loves, loves, loves stewed dried fruit. With the nutrients concentrated with drying of fruit, this simple dessert is not only yummy, but packed with nutrients . . . and cooking the fruits lessens the effects of sugar, so it couldn't be more perfect.

4-5 dried apricots, pitted
3-4 dried prunes, pitted
½ cup dried cherries, pitted
½ cup raisins
pinch sea salt
½ cup dry white wine
2 teaspoons honey
grated zest of 1 lemon
2-3 tablespoons slivered almonds

Place all ingredients in a sauce pan over medium heat, cover and bring to a boil. Reduce heat to low and cook until fruit is quite soft and liquid has thickened, about 20 minutes.

To serve, spoon fruit into individual dessert cups and sprinkle with almonds. Makes 3-4 servings.

Steamed Cranberry-Apple Pudding

Talk about having your cake and eating it too. For many people with bone trouble, hard baked flour can exacerbate their symptoms and discomfort. But rather than doom them a life of no treats, give this delicate steamed pudding a whirl . . . nutritious, sweet and moist, this traditional dessert is a real winner.

2 cups whole wheat pastry flour
½ cup semolina flour
3 teaspoons baking powder
pinch sea salt
scant pinch cinnamon
½ cup light olive or avocado oil
1 teaspoon pure vanilla extract
½ cup brown rice syrup or honey
2/3-1 cup vanilla soymilk
½ cup unsweetened dried cranberries
1 small Granny Smith apple, seeded, diced (do not peel)
¼ cup finely diced pecan pieces

Lightly oil a 3-quart pudding basin and its lid.

Whisk together flours, baking powder, salt and cinnamon. Mix in oil, vanilla and sweetener. Slowly mix in soymilk to create a smooth, spoonable batter. Fold in cranberries, apples and nuts. Spoon batter into prepared pudding basin, cover, seal and place in a large pot. Add water to half cover pudding basin, cover and bring to a boil. Reduce heat to low and cook for 2 hours, occasionally checking the water amount, adding as needed to keep it half covering the basin.

After 2 hours, carefully remove pudding basin from steaming water and allow to stand, undisturbed, for 10 minutes. Remove cover and invert pudding onto a serving plate. Serve warm or at room temperature. This pudding is lovely served with stewed fruit. Makes 5-6 servings.

Note: You can pressure cook the pudding and shorten cooking time by 1 hour. Follow the same cooking directions, but cook for only 1 hour under full pressure.

Gratin of Red and Black Berries

What? Gratin? Those dairy and sugar filled decadent treats? How can we make one of those and have them be healthy for us? Simple . . . this recipe. Tannin and polyphenol-rich berries smothered in a creamy sauce and baked to sweet perfection . . .

2 cups vanilla soymilk
2 teaspoons kuzu or arrowroot, dissolved in a small amount of cold water
1 teaspoon pure vanilla extract
pinch sea salt
1 cup raspberries, rinsed well
1 cup blackberries, rinsed well
1 cup blueberries, rinsed well
2-3 tablespoons maple granules
1-2 sprigs fresh mint

Preheat oven to 325o and lightly oil a 1-quart shallow baking dish.

Place soymilk, vanilla and salt in a sauce pan over low heat. When the soymilk is warmed through, stir in dissolved kuzu and cook, stirring constantly, until the mixture thickens, about 3 minutes. Set aside to cool slightly, stirring frequently so it doesn't set.

Arrange berries in the prepared baking dish. Spoon soymilk mixture over the berries, filling the dish completely. Sprinkle generously with maple granules and bake until the granules have melted and the berries are bubbling, 15-20 minutes. Remove form oven and allow to stand for 10 minutes before serving.

To serve, scoop into individual dessert cups and garnish with fresh mint, if desired. Makes 3-4 servings.

Apple Crumble

Another favorite of my husband. He love simple, cozy and homey desserts, nothing fancy. In this, we showcase the wonders of apples . . . filled with vitamins and minerals essential to our well-being, but in particular, pectin, a compound that helps to keep our cholesterol in check. And the fact that it's yummy is just icing on the cake, so to speak.

filling:
3-4 ripe apples, like gala, Macintosh or granny smith, seeded, diced, do not
    peel
½ cup golden raisins
scant pinch cinnamon
pinch sea salt
2-3 tablespoons arrowroot
3 tablespoons light olive or avocado oil

crumble:
1 cup walnut or pecan pieces, coarsely chopped
¼ cup whole wheat pastry flour
pinch sea salt
¼ cup light olive or avocado oil
½ cup brown rice syrup or honey
vanilla soymilk

Preheat oven to 350o.
    Place apples and raisins in a bowl. Add balance of ingredients and toss to coat. Spoon filling into a shallow baking dish.
    Make the topping. Combine nuts, flour and salt in a mixing bowl. Stir in oil and sweetener. Slowly add soymilk until a crumbly, moist texture forms.
    Spoon topping over apples, covering, but letting the fruit peek through. Cover and bake for 20 minutes. Remove cover and bake until topping is golden and crisp and fruit is soft, about 15 minutes. Makes 4-5 servings.

Berry Crisp

Tanins and polyphenols are compounds in foods that help us maintain our health . . . from our organ function to immune function to brain function to our bone density. These compounds, concentrated in brightly colored foods, like berries, are some of the most important keys to our well-being.

filling:
2 cups blueberries, sorted, rinsed well
1 cup raspberries, rinsed well
1 cup blackberries, rinsed well
1 cup diced strawberries
grated zest of 1 fresh lemon
pinch sea salt
¼ cup light olive or avocado oil
2 tablespoons honey
2 tablespoons arrowroot

crisp:
1 cup coarsely chopped pecan pieces
pinch sea salt
4 tablespoons light olive or avocado oil
scant pinch nutmeg
1/3 cup maple granules

Preheat oven to 350o and lightly oil a shallow baking dish.

Place berries in a mixing bowl and add balance of ingredients. Gently stir to coat fruit, taking care not to break the berries. Spread evenly in baking dish.

Make the topping by combining all ingredients and mixing very well to create a crumbly texture. Sprinkle topping over fruit, covering abundantly. Cover and bake for 15 minutes. Remove cover and bake until topping is crisp and golden and the fruit is bubbling, about 15 minutes. Makes 5-6 servings.

Baked Apricots with Almond Cream

Apricots are not only some of the most luscious fruits that summer gifts to us, but some of the most nutrient-dense. Rich in iron, magnesium, potassium and vitamin C, these jewels are as good as they are good for us.

almond cream:
1 cup almond milk
1 teaspoon honey
pinch sea salt
1 tablespoons agar flakes
1 tablespoon kuzu, dissolved in small amount of cold water
4 ripe apricots, halved lengthwise, stones removed, do not peel
extra virgin olive oil

pinch sea salt
4 tablespoons honey
3 tablespoons slivered almonds, lightly pan toasted

Preheat oven to 350o and line a baking sheet with parchment.

Make the almond crème by combining almond milk, honey, salt and agar in a sauce pan over low heat. Stir well and cook over low heat until agar is dissolved, about 20 minutes. Stir in dissolved kuzu and cook, stirring until the mixture thickens, about 4 minutes. Transfer to a heat-resistant bowl and set aside for 15 minutes. Place in the refrigerator to set.

While the almond crème cooks, place the apricots, cut side up, on the lined baking sheet. Drizzle with oil, add a sprinkle of salt and drizzle honey over fruit. Bake until fruit is tender enough to pierce with a fork, about 25 minutes.

When the almond crème is set, whip to a creamy texture in a food processor or with a hand blender.

To serve, place apricot halves on individual serving plates, with a dollop of almond crème on top. Sprinkle with slivered almonds and serve. Makes 4-8 servings.

Apple Tart

A cozier dessert is not to be had . . . autumn's freshest apples, crisp and lush, nestled in a flaky pastry crust and topped with a crunchy streusel . . . yum. And with pectin from apples and omega 3 from hempseeds keeping our blood strong and vital, it's the perfect dessert.

pastry:
1 cup whole wheat pastry flour
½ cup semolina flour
pinch sea salt
¼ cup light olive or avocado oil
spring or filtered water

filling:
extra virgin olive oil
6-8 firm apples, gala, Macintosh, granny smith, fuji, seeded, thinly sliced, do not peel
pinch sea salt
scant pinch cinnamon
grated zest of 1 lemon
2-3 tablespoons brown rice syrup or honey

streusel:
2/3 cup coarsely chopped pecan pieces
1/3 cup unsweetened shredded coconut
1 tablespoon shelled hempseeds
pinch sea salt
scant pinch cinnamon
1/3 cup maple granules
¼-1/3 cup light olive or avocado oil

Preheat oven to 350o and lightly oil a 12-inch tart pan with removable bottom.

Make the crust by combining flours and salt in a mixing bowl. Using a fork or a pastry cutter, cut the oil into the flour, creating the texture of wet sand. Slowly add water to create a soft, rollable crust. Gather into a ball, wrap in plastic and set aside to rest for 10 minutes. Roll into a thin round, about an inch larger than the tart pan. Lay the crust on the pan and fit it into the crevices, without stretching the dough. Trim the excess flush with the rim. Pierce in several places with a fork.

Make the filling by placing a small amount of oil in a deep skillet over medium heat. Sauté apples with a pinch of salt and cinnamon for 2 minutes. Add lemon zest and honey and sauté for 2 minutes more. Set aside to cool to warm.

While the apples cool, make the streusel. Combine all ingredients, mixing until the texture is crumbly.

Spoon apples into tart shell. Sprinkle streusel topping over the filling, covering completely. Cover loosely with foil and bake for 25 minutes. Remove cover and bake until crust is lightly browned, streusel is crisp and apples are quite tender, about 35 minutes more. Remove from oven and allow to cool for 10 minutes before removing from tart pan and slicing into wedges. Makes 8-10 servings.

Blueberry-Plum Galette

This country tart is not only easy to make and delicious to eat, but incredibly nutritious. With the tannins in blueberries keeping our minds sharp and the iron, calcium and vitamin C in the plums keeping our blood and bones strong, this is a dessert fit for a king.

galette crust:
1 cup whole wheat pastry flour
½ cup semolina flour
½ teaspoon baking powder

pinch sea salt
¼ cup light olive or avocado oil
spring or filtered water

filling:
2 cups fresh blueberries, sorted, rinsed well
2-3 fresh plums, halved, seeded, diced, do not peel
¼ cup light olive or avocado oil
¼ cup brown rice syrup or honey
scant pinch nutmeg
grated zest of ½ lemon
3 tablespoons arrowroot

Preheat oven to 350o and line a round pizza tin with parchment.

Make the crust by combining flours with baking powder and salt. Using a fork or pastry cutter, cut in oil to create the texture of wet sand. Slowly add water, mixing until you create a firm, rollable texture. Gather into a ball and wrap in plastic. Set aside for 15 minutes.

Make the filling by simply combining all ingredients in a mixing bowl and tossing to coat.

Lightly flour a flat dry surface and roll out dough to create a round that is about 1/8-inch thick. Spoon filling into the center of the dough. Spread it toward the edges, leaving about 2 inches of dough exposed. Fold dough up over filling, leaving the filling exposed in the center. Press the dough to form pleats over the filling, but be sure that the center is open.

Bake until the filling is bubbling and the crust is lightly golden and firm to the touch, 35-40 minutes. Makes 6-8 servings.

Strawberry-Raspberry Tart

Oh, man . . . summer just ain't summer 'til I make this tart. Just when the strawberries are in and the weather is warming my winter-weary skin. And with vitamin C, tannins, polyphenols, folic acid and vitamin D, berries are one of summer's greatest gifts to our health.

tart crust:
1 cup whole wheat pastry flour
½ cup semolina flour
scant pinch cinnamon
pinch sea salt

¼ cup light olive or avocado oil
spring or filtered water

filling:
2 cups sliced fresh strawberries
2 cups fresh raspberries, sorted, rinsed well
pinch sea salt
3 tablespoons honey
grated zest of ½ lemon
2 tablespoons light olive or avocado oil
2 tablespoons arrowroot
1 cup slivered almonds

Preheat oven to 350o and lightly oil a 12-inch tart pan with removable bottom.

Make the crust by combining flours and salt in a mixing bowl. Using a fork or a pastry cutter, cut the oil into the flour, creating the texture of wet sand. Slowly add water to create a soft, rollable crust. Gather into a ball, wrap in plastic and set aside to rest for 10 minutes. Roll into a thin round, about an inch larger than the tart pan. Lay the crust on the pan and fit it into the crevices, without stretching the dough. Trim the excess flush with the rim. Pierce in several places with a fork.

Make the filling by placing berries in a mixing bowl with the balance of ingredients. Toss gently to coat, taking care not to break the berries. Spoon filling evenly into shell. Sprinkle with almonds and cover loosely. Bake for 15 minutes. Remove cover and bake until crust is golden and filling is bubbling, 20 minutes more. Remove from oven and allow to stand for 10 minutes before removing from tart pan and slicing into wedges. Makes 6-8 servings.

Double Crust Cherry Pie

When cherries are in season, it's hard to make this pie, because I keep eating the cherries before I can get them pitted and into the mixing bowl. But try to restrain yourself. It'll be worth it for this pie. With polyphenols, vitamin C, iron, magnesium, potassium and folic acid, these babies are great for our health . . . and in a pie? With flaky crust? Yum.

crust:
2 cups whole wheat pastry flour
1 cup semolina flour
pinch sea salt

1/2 cup light olive or avocado oil
spring or filtered water

filling:
light olive oil
4 cups fresh cherries, pitted
pinch sea salt
3 tablespoons brown rice syrup of honey
grated zest of ½ lemon
3 tablespoons arrowroot

Preheat oven to 325o and lightly oil a standard deep dish pie plate.

Make the crust by combining flours and salt in a mixing bowl. Using a fork or a pastry cutter, cut the oil into the flour, creating the texture of wet sand. Slowly add water to create a soft, rollable crust. Gather into a ball, wrap in plastic and set aside to rest for 10 minutes. Roll half the dough into a thin round, about an inch larger than the tart pan. Lay the crust on the pie plate and fit it in, without stretching the dough. Trim the excess to allow for a slight overhang. Roll the other half of the dough into a round the size of the pie plate. Pierce bottom crust in several places with a fork.

Make the filling by placing all ingredients in a sauce pan over low heat. Cook for 5-7 minutes. Remove from heat and cool for 10 minutes. Stir in arrowroot, tossing to coat the cherries. Spoon filling into pie plate. Lay top crust over filling. Pull edges of bottom crust up over the rim of the top crust. Pleat decoratively to seal the rim of the crust. Using a sharp knife, make deep slits in the top crust to allow steam to escape.

Place pie on a sheet pan and lay a foil tent over top. Bake for 25 minutes. Remove cover and bake for another 35-40 minutes, until the crust is lightly browned and firm to the touch. Remove from heat and allow to stand for 10 minutes before slicing into wedges. Makes 8-10 servings.

Spiced Apple Cake

A homey, sweet delicate cake, laced through with crisp apples and perfectly spiced to enhance the apple flavor . . . and aid in the digestion of the dessert . . . pretty perfect, yes?

2 ½ cups whole wheat pastry flour
½ cup semolina flour
generous pinch sea salt
3 teaspoons baking powder

scant pinch cinnamon
scant pinch nutmeg
scant pinch dried thyme
½ cup light olive or avocado oil
½ cup honey
1 teaspoon pure vanilla extract
½-1 cup vanilla soymilk
2 Granny Smith apples, seeded, diced, do not peel
1/3 cup coarsely chopped walnut pieces

lemon glaze:
½ cup honey
pinch sea salt
grated zest of ½ lemon

Preheat oven to 350o and lightly oil and flour a standard bundt pan.

Whisk together flours, salt, baking powder and spices. Mix in oil, honey and vanilla. Slowly mix in soymilk to create a smooth, spoonable cake batter. Fold in apples and walnuts. Spoon batter into prepared pan and bake until the top of the cake springs back to the touch, about 45 minutes.

Remove from heat and allow to stand, undisturbed, for 10 minutes before inverting cake onto a serving plate.

Make the glaze by combining ingredients in a sauce pan over medium heat. When the honey foams, simply spoon over cake, allowing glaze to run down the sides of the cake. Slice into wedges. Makes 8-10 servings.

Peach Upside Down Cake

Summer peaches are such a blessing, such a treat. We can never eat enough of them, right? Out of hand, in compotes, on cereal . . . well, here's a new idea for you . . . one that will become a regular part of your summer menu plans.

4 tablespoons light olive or avocado oil
4 tablespoons brown rice syrup or honey
grated zest of ½ lemon
pinch sea salt
4 ripe peaches, halved lengthwise, stones removed, peeled

cake:
2 cups whole wheat pastry flour
½ cup semolina flour

pinch sea salt
3 teaspoons baking powder
1/3 cup light olive or avocado oil
1/3 cup brown rice syrup or honey
1 teaspoon pure vanilla extract
½-2/3 cup vanilla soymilk

Preheat oven to 350o.

Place a 13-inch cast iron skillet with oil, sweetener, lemon zest and salt over medium heat. Cook, while stirring, for 2 minutes. Lay peach halves, cut-side down, in the mixture and reduce heat to low. Cook while preparing the cake batter.

Make the batter by whisking together flours, salt and baking powder. Mix in oil, sweetener and vanilla. Slowly add soymilk, stirring constantly, to create a smooth spoonable batter. Remove skillet from heat. Carefully spoon batter over the cooked peaches, taking care not to disturb peaches. Place skillet in the oven and bake until the top of the cake springs back to the touch, 40-45 minutes. Remove from heat and allow to stand for 10 minutes before inverting cake onto a serving plate. If any of the peaches stick to the pan, simply scoop out of the skillet and replace on the cake. Spoon remaining glaze over the cake. Slice into wedges. Makes 6-8 servings.

Almond Fruitcake

Before you skip this recipe . . . you know what I mean . . . oh, no . . . the fruitcake recipe! This one is moist, hearty and laced through with nutrient-packed dried fruit, from apricots to raisins, with everything from calcium to magnesium to iron to omega-3 . . . trust me, you won't re-gift this fruitcake.

2 cups whole wheat pastry flour
½ cup semolina flour
3 teaspoons baking powder
pinch sea salt
scant pinch cinnamon
scant pinch nutmeg
scant pinch cardoman
1/3 cup light olive or avocado oil
½ cup honey
1 teaspoon pure vanilla extract
½-1 cup vanilla soymilk
3-4 dried apricots, soaked until tender, diced
3-4 dried prunes, soaked until tender, diced
3-4 dried apples, soaked until tender, diced

3-4 dried pears, soaked until tender, diced
¼ cup raisins
½ cup almond meal*

Preheat oven to 350o and lightly oil and flour a standard bundt pan.

Whisk together flours, baking powder, salt and spices. Mix in oil, honey and vanilla. Slowly stir in soymilk to create a smooth, pourable batter. Fold in fruit and almond meal. Spoon batter evenly into prepared pan and bake until the top of the cake springs back to the touch, 45-50 minutes. Remove from oven and allow to stand 10 minutes before inverting onto a serving plate. Slice into wedges. Makes 8-10 servings.

You can either purchase almond meal or grind blanched almonds into fine meal in a food processor.

Oatmeal Cranberry Cookies

Oatmeal cookies are some of the most delicious, familiar cookies, but the ones we buy are laced through with simple sugar that can rob our bones of precious minerals. So . . . make a batch of these . . . and in place of raisins, try dried cranberries to add some delicate tartness.

1 cup whole wheat pastry flour
½ cup rolled oats
pinch sea salt
1 teaspoon baking powder
scant pinch cinnamon
¼ cup unsweetened shredded coconut
¼ cup light olive or avocado oil
½ cup brown rice syrup
1 teaspoon pure vanilla extract
vanilla soymilk
1/3 cup dried, unsweetened cranberries
1/3 cup coarsely chopped pecan pieces

Preheat oven to 350o and line a baking sheet with parchment.

Mix together flour, oats, salt, baking powder, cinnamon and coconut. Mix in oil, rice syrup and vanilla with enough soymilk to create a spoonable batter. Fold in cranberries and pecans.

Drop, by tablespoons, onto lined baking sheet, leaving about an inch between cookies. Bake for 18 minutes. Remove from oven and allow to cool on baking sheet for 2 minutes. Transfer to a wire rack and cool completely. Makes about 24 cookies.

Banana Chocolate Chip Cookies

Not just any chocolate chip cookies, we add bananas for moisture, sweet taste and precious potassium for our health. Now that's food of the gods.

2 cups whole wheat pastry flour
½ cup semolina flour
pinch sea salt
1 teaspoon baking powder
scant pinch cinnamon
1/3 cup light olive or avocado oil
1/3 cup honey
1 teaspoon pure vanilla extract
1 very ripe banana, mashed
vanilla soymilk
2/3 cup non-dairy, grain-sweetened chocolate chips
1/3 cup coarsely chopped pecan pieces

Preheat oven to 350o and line a baking sheet with parchment.

Mix flours, salt, baking powder and cinnamon together. Mix in oil, honey and vanilla. Mix in banana. Slowly add soymilk to create a spoonable batter. Fold in chocolate chips and pecans.

Drop by spoonfuls onto lined sheet and bake for 18-20 minutes, until cookies are firm at the edges and soft in the centers. Remove from oven and allow cookies to cool on sheet for 2 minutes. Transfer to a wire rack and cool completely. Make about 24 cookies.

Raspberry Bars

Bar cookies are just yummy and so easy to make, there's no excuse to eat junk and white sugar. In these, we use raspberries for the tannins and polyphenols for our well-being and vitality.

bars:
2 cups whole wheat pastry flour
½ cup semolina flour
pinch sea salt

1 teaspoon baking powder
¼ cup unsweetened shredded coconut
scant pinch cardoman
1/3 cup light olive or avocado oil
1/3 cup brown rice syrup
1 teaspoon pure vanilla extract
vanilla soymilk
2/3 cup finely chopped walnut pieces

filling:
½ cup unsweetened raspberry preserves
½ cup brown rice syrup
grated zest of ½ lemon

Preheat oven to 350o and lightly oil a 9-inch square glass baking dish.

Prepare batter by mixing together all dry ingredients. Mix in oil, rice syrup and vanilla. Slowly stir in soymilk to create a stiff, but spoonable batter.

Make the filling by mixing ingredients together.

Spread half the batter over the bottom of the baking dish. Spoon filling over the batter, covering completely. Spoon remaining batter over the filling, covering completely. Bake until the filling is bubbling and the topping is firm to the touch, 30-35 minutes. Remove from oven and allow to cool for 10 minutes before cutting into squares. Makes 8-12 servings.

Almond Biscotti

These double-baked crisp cookies are just the best for dipping in strong espresso . . . or tea for the more delicate of heart. Cocoa powder, chocolate chips and dipped in chocolate glaze, these yummy cookies are a chocolate lovers dream.

1 2/3 cups whole wheat pastry flour
1/3 cup semolina flour
1/3 cup unsweetened cocoa powder
2 teaspoons baking powder
generous pinch sea salt
scant pinch ground cinnamon
1/3 cup hempseed or light olive oil
cup brown rice syrup
1 teaspoon pure vanilla extract
vanilla soymilk
½ cup slivered almonds

ganache:
1 cup non-dairy, grain-sweetened chocolate chips
2 teaspoons brown rice syrup
1/4 cup vanilla soymilk

Preheat oven to 350o and line a baking sheet with parchment.

Whisk together flours, cocoa powder, baking powder, salt and cinnamon. Mix in oil, rice syrup and vanilla, stirring to combine. Slowly add soymilk to create a soft, pliable dough. Knead 2-3 times to hold batter together. Fold in almonds to incorporate them into the dough. Divide dough in half and, with moist hands, form each half into a long log about 10 inches long and 2 inches wide. Bake until the top of each log is firm, 30-35 minutes. Remove from oven and allow to stand, on the baking sheet for 2 minutes. Carefully transfer each log to a dry cutting board, and using a sharp, serrated knife, slice each long into 3/4-inch-thick slices. Lay the slices, cut-side up on the baking sheet and bake for 3 minutes. Turn the slices so the other cut side is up and bake for 3-4 minutes, so cookies are crisp. Remove from oven and allow to cool on the baking sheet.

Once the biscotti have cooled completely, make the ganache. Place the chocolate chips in a heat-resistant bowl. Combine rice syrup and soymilk in a small sauce pan and bring to a rolling boil over high heat. Pour over chocolate and whisk to form a smooth shiny ganache.

Dip one half of each biscotti and place on parchment. Allow to stand until glaze sets. You can also place the ganache in a squeeze bottle and drizzle chocolate over each cookie. Makes 24-30 biscotti.

Note: Hempseed oil is high in an albumin-like protein (like eggs) and helps to prevent the biscotti from crumbling when slicing.

Apricot Kiss Cookies

A wonderful cookie that I make in the summer, to celebrate apricots. At their freshest best in hot weather, apricots are sweet, sensual and richly satisfying with little enhancement. The sweet filling is encased in a soft pastry, making for the perfect sweet treat.

pastry:
2 cups whole wheat pastry flour
generous pinch sea salt
teaspoon baking powder
pinch cinnamon
1/4 cup avocado or light olive oil vanilla soymilk

filling:
20-24 fresh apricots, split, stones removed, coarsely chopped
3 tablespoons brown rice syrup
pinch sea salt
grated zest of 1 lemon
2-3 tablespoons vanilla soymilk
1-2 tablespoons kuzu, dissolved in small amount cold water

Preheat oven to 350o and line a baking sheet with parchment.

Make the pastry by whisking together flour, salt, baking powder and cinnamon. Cut in oil with a fork or a pastry cutter to create the texture of crumbling sand. Slowly mix in soymilk to create a soft, pliable dough, not too sticky or too dry. Knead 2-3 times to gather the dough into a ball. Wrap in plastic and set aside.

Prepare the filling by combining apricots, rice syrup, salt, lemon zest and soymilk in a saucepan and turning the heat to medium-low. Cook, stirring frequently until the apricots are soft, about 15 minutes. Stir in dissolved kuzu and cook, stirring, until the mixture thickens, about 3 minutes.

Roll out dough between two sheets of parchment creating a rectangle of dough that is about 1/8-inch thick. Using a 3-inch cookie cutter or glass, cut round shapes in the dough. Place a teaspoon of filling on one side of each round, fold over, creating a half moon. Seal the edges of each half moon with a fork, pressing them together to create a decorative edge. Place each apricot kiss on the lined baking sheet. Repeat with remaining ingredients, re-rolling dough as necessary.

Bake apricot kisses until they are firm to the touch and edges are lightly browned, 20-28 minutes. Remove from oven and transfer to a wire rack to cool completely. Makes 20-24 cookies.

Note: For added zip, cook some rice syrup to a high foam and spoon it over each cookie as a sticky glaze.

Resource Directory

For many, some of the information and recipe ingredients referenced in this book may seem foreign or exotic. If you have questions, or require additional information on any of the products referenced in this book, contact:

Christina Cooks
243 Dickinson Street
Philadelphia, PA 19147-6003
1-800-939-3909

You may also visit our website: www.christinacooks.com

About the Authors

Robert Pirello

Robert Pirello hails from Boston, Massachusetts and has one ambition in life . . . to run The Boston Marathon on his 100th birthday. His commitment to living a healthy lifestyle may be just the ticket to making that dream a reality. On his way to his 100th birthday, Robert has worked in marketing, advertising, and public relations for all of his professional life.

Robert is a graduate of Northeast School of Communications, and Leland Powers School of theatre, both in Boston Massachusetts, where he studied broadcast communications, journalism, and theatrical arts. Robert studied marketing through the Bank Marketing Institute; and alternative health at The Kushi Institute in Boston, Massachusetts.

Starting out in radio, Robert has worked in the advertising business from every angle, with experience as both the client and the agency, giving him a 'Renaissance man' style of understanding of how advertising, marketing, and public relations works. As the client, Robert worked for his companies to best market their financial services and as the agency, Robert has worked with some of the best creative talent in print, radio, television production, trade show exhibits and other media outlets.

As well as a strong marketing background, Robert brings a deep understanding of alternative health and the natural foods industry to the table. Robert has researched and studied most every aspect of alternative health. A pioneer in the soy foods industry, in the early 1980's, Robert worked as the creator and manufacturer of the first non-dairy soy-based cheese. This successful business gave Robert a wisdom and understanding that can only come with hard work and experience.

Today, as executive producer of the nationally broadcast public television series 'Christina Cooks,' Robert has brought all his years of experience, as well as his insightful vision to steer the creation of this successful alternative, 'healthy', cooking show and related enterprises. His understanding of alternative health, and the natural foods industry allows for a deep understanding of what is important to the consumer, and how best to communicate that message. All his skills combine to create the driving force behind the enterprise that is 'Christina Cooks.'

Oh, Robert has one other ambition . . . to live in Tuscany, driving a small Italian car with the license plate 'XAd Man'.

Bernardo A Merizalde, MD

Bernardo Merizalde was born in White Plains, NY and moved to Colombia, South America, at the age of three years old, where he was raised and educated. Bernardo is a graduate of the medical school at the Universidad de Rosario, in Bogota, which was founded in the 18th century. There, he learned patient management and treatment by doing it, since interns and residents were not a common occurrence.

By the last year of medical school, Bernardo saw the limitations of conventional medicine and decided to explore alternative approaches. Beginning with acupuncture and herbal medicine, Bernardo later became interested in homeopathic medicine. He did part of his medical internship in the jungles of Colombia, but did not apprentice with any shaman! Bernardo then began integrating the alternative/complementary approaches into his practice of general medicine, which he has practiced for more than twenty-five years.

Moving to Philadelphia, Pennsylvania, in the United States, Bernardo attended Hahnemann Hospital's Psychiatry and Neurology residency program and became Board Certified. Hahnemann Hospital was originally a homeopathic hospital. Bernardo found that learning about the mind and mind-body relationships helped him to become a better rounded practitioner, giving him tools to address the emotional and spiritual components of healing.

Currently, Bernardo practices general medicine and psychiatry in Lafayette Hill, Pennsylvania; gives lectures to various local medical schools as an invited guest, and is an officer of the Board of Directors of the American Institute of Homeopathy, the oldest extant medical organization in the US.

Bernardo believes the key solution to our human problems, social, economic and political, is an improvement in physical, emotional and mental health.

Christina Pirello

Christina Pirello, Emmy Award-winning host of the television series, 'Christina Cooks', is a bright, free-spirited, vivacious redhead who found her way to Philadelphia by opening a map and dropping a pin. Her relationship with food began early, cooking with her mother and later, while she was living in Florida, working as a caterer and pastry chef. But the real pivotal point in her life came at age 26, when after being diagnosed with terminal leukemia, she decided to forego conventional medical therapies and turned to a nutritional approach to cure herself. The passion and commitment which made that happen is what makes her so wonderfully inspirational at what she does today.

In 1997 she launched 'Christina Cooks', her popular, nationally broadcast public television series. 'Christina Cooks' is a half-hour of amazing thought-provoking, fun and practical information about food, beauty and lifestyle. In 2000, CN8, The Comcast Network, contracted with Christina to broadcast her show as well. Christina, who since 1983, has been teaching whole foods cooking, conducting lifestyle seminars and lecturing on the power of food, challenges us to create a whole new relationship with the food we eat. From corporate boardrooms to network TV, Christina inspires her audiences and viewers to take control of their lives through their diet. 'Christina Cooks' has also found its way into the hearts and kitchens of a worldwide audience through Christina's books and international distribution on the Discovery Health Network.

For over twenty years, Christina has been teaching whole foods cooking classes, conducting lifestyle seminars and lecturing on the power of food in our lives nationwide, in a variety of settings. No lives are left unchanged when she leaves the room. Even if people think she's nuts (but nice), they'll never think of food in the same way again . . . which is her goal. The author of the best-selling cookbook, *Cooking the Whole Foods Way*, Christina has also released *Cook Your Way to the Life You Want*, *GLOW, A Prescription for Radiant Health and Beauty*; and *Christina Cooks, Everything You Ever Wanted to Know About Whole Foods but Were Afraid to Ask*, all published by H.P. Books, a division of Penguin Group (USA) Inc.

Having won an Emmy Award in the category of 'Best Host', Christina is regularly featured in newspapers and magazines, as well as on TV and radio, Christina has been featured in: Prevention Magazine; Newsweek; Seventeen; Natural Health; Natural Healing; and Women First. She has been seen on The CBS Early Show; NBC's The Other Half with Dick Clark; Home Matters on The Discovery Channel; Women's Day TV on The PAX TV Network; and The TV Food Network.

In addition, Christina is on the faculty of Drexel University, and holds a Masters degree in nutrition.

References and Bibliography

Adinoff AD & Hollister JR, "Steroid induced fracture and bone loss in patients with asthma, New England Journal of Medicine, 309 (5), 265-268.

Agency for Healthcare Research and Quality. Recommendations and rationale: screening for osteoporosis in postmenopausal women. US Preventive Task Force. Guide to Clinical Preventive Services. 3rd ed. 2002. Available at: http://www. ahrq.gov/clinic/3rduspstf/osteoporosis/osteorr.htm Accessed December 22, 2003.

Apgar BS. HRT dilemma. Program and abstracts of the American Academy of Family Physicians 2003 Annual Scientific Assembly; October 1-5, 2003; New Orleans, Louisiana. Abstract 12.

AAFP, American Academy of Family Physicians: Osteoporosis. Recommendations for Periodic Health Examinations. Clinical Care & Research, *http://www.aafp. org/x24974.xml Accessed 1/27/04.*

Azria M,"The value of biomarkers in detecting alterations in bone metabolism", Calcif Tissue Int.1989;45:7-11.

Bartsch H, Bartsch C, "Effect of melatonin in experimental tumors under different photoperiods and times of administration, J Neural Transm, 52; 269-279, 1981.

Bartsch C, Bartsch H, et al, "Depleted pineal melatonin production in primary breast and prostate cancer is connected with circadian disturbances: possible role of melatonin for synchronization of circadian rhythmicity. In: Touitou Y, Arendt J, Pevet P, eds., "Melatonin and the Pineal Gland—From Basic Science to Clinical Application", New York, NY, Elseview, 311-316, 1993.

Bellavite, P. (2003). Complexity science and homeopathy: a synthetic overview. Homeopathy: the Journal of the Faculty of Homeopathy. 92, 203-212 Biological Sulfur and Your Health, www.nutriteam.com/msm.htm

Bischoff HA, Staehelin HB, Dick W, et al. Fall prevention by vitamin D and calcium supplementation: a randomised controlled trial. J Bone Miner Res. 2001;16(suppl 1):S163.

Brown S. "Better Bones, Better Body: Beyond Estrogen and Calcium", Los Angeles: Keats Publishing, 1996.

Campbell TC. et al, "Diet and Health in Rural China: Lessons Learned and Unlearned", Nutrition Today, 34:3 (1999) 116-23.

Cann C, et al, "Decreased spinal mineral content in amenorrheic women, Journal of the American Medical Association, 251 (5), 626-629, 1984.

Carman JS, Post RM, et al, "Negative effects of melatonin on depression", American Journal Psychiatry, 133: 1181-1186, 1976.

Cell Tech International, www.celltech.com

Center for Disease Control, Savannah River Site Health Effects Subcommittee Meeting, January 2002. http//cdc.gov/nceh/radiation/savannah/SRSHES_Toxicity_jan02.htm. (Accessed Aug. 2004)

Chestnut CH, Silverman S, Andriano K, et al. A randomized trial of nasal spray salmon calcitonin in post-menopausal women with established osteoporosis: the prevention of recurrence of osteoporotic fractures study. PROOF Study Group. Am J Med. 2000;109:267-276.

Chiu KC, et al, "**Hypovitaminosis D is associated with insulin resistance and ß cell dysfunction** Am J Clin Nutr 2004;79:820-825.

Choosing Health Oils, www.cybreezes.com

Conly J, Stein K. Reduction of vitamin K2 concentrations in human liver associated with the use of broad spectrum antimicrobials. Clin Invest Med 1994 Dec;17(6):531-9

Comprehensive Anti-aging Research, *www.qualitycounts.com*, osteoporosis

Cumming RG, et al, "Case Control Study of risk Factors for Hip Fractures in the Elderly", American Journal of Epidemiology 139 (19940 493-503.

Cummings SR, Nevitt MC, Browner WS, et al, Risk factors of hip fracture in white women, Study of Steoporotic Risk Factors Research Group, N. Eng. J of Med 1995; 332 (12) 767-73.

Daniels, D, "Exercise for Osteoporosis", Hatherleigh Press, 2000.

Delmas PD. Clinical use of biochemical markers of bone remodeling in osteoporosis", Bone 1992;13:S17-21.

Delmas PD et al. "Urinary excretion of pyridinoline crosslinks correlates with bone turnover measured on iliac crest biopsy in patients with vertebral osteoporosis", J Bone Min Res 1991;6(6):639-44.

Dhore CR, Cleutjens JP, Lutgens E, et. al. Differential expression of bone matrix regulatory proteins in human atherosclerotic plaques. Arterioscler Thromb Vasc Biol. 2001 Dec;21(12):1998-2003

Eaton S, et al, "Calcium in evolutionary perspective", American Journal of Clinical Nutrition, 54 (suppl.), 281S-287S.

Elia, V., Niccoli, M. (1999). Thermodynamics of extremely diluted aqueous solutions. Annals of the New York Academy of Sciences 879, 241-248.

Elia, V., Niccoli, M. (2004). New physico-chemical properties of extremely diluted aqueous solutions. Journal of Thermal Analysis and Calorimetry 75, 815-836.

Ettinger B., "An update for the obstetriciangynecologist on advances in the diagnosis, prevention, and treatment of postmenopausal osteoporosis", Current Opinion OB G.YN 1993;5:396-403.

Feskanich D, et al, "Milk Dietary Calcium, and Bone Fractures in Women . . .", American Journal of Public Health 87 (1997) 992-7.

Forsling ML, Williams AJ, "The effects exogenous melatonin on stimulated neurohypophyseal hormone release in man", Clin Endocrinol (Oxf), 57, 615-620, 2002.

Franklin JA, et al, "Long term thyroxin treatment and bone mineral density, Lancet, 340, 9-13, 1992.

Gaby AR, "Preventing and Reversing Osteoporosis", Prima Publishing, 1996.

Garber AK, Binkley NC, Krueger DC, et. al. Comparison of phylloquinone bioavailability from food sources or a supplement in human subjects. J Nutr. 1999 Jun;129(6):1201-3.

Germano, C, "The Osteoporosis Solution", Kensington Health, 1999.

Gold PW, et al, "Responses to corticotrophin-releasing hormone in the hypercortisolism of drepssion and Cushing's disease: Pathophysiological and diagnostic implications. New England Journal of Medicine, 314, 1329-1335, 1986.

Grady D, Herrington D, Bittner V, et al, for the HERS Research Group. Cardiovascular disease outcomes during 6.8 years of hormone therapy: Heart and Estrogen/progesterone Replacement Study Follow-up (HERS II). JAMA. 2002;288:58-66.

Great Smokies Diagnostic Laboratories, www.gsdl.com, 2004.

Guyton & Hall, Textbook of Medical Physiology, Tenth Edition, W.B.Saunders, Philadelphia, 2000.

Hahneman S.1842/1996: "Organon of Medicine," Translation of the sixth edition by Wenda Brewster O'Reilly, Birdcage Books, Redmond, WA.

Harris W, "The Scientific Basis of Vegetarianism", second printing, Hawaii Health Publishers, Honolulu, HI, 1996.

Hassager C et al., "Effect of menopause and hormone replacement therapy on urinary excretion of pyridinium cross-sectional study", Clin Endocrinology 1992;37:45-50.

Heaney, RP, Recker RR, "Effects of Nitrogen, Phosphorus, and Caffeine on Calcium balance in women", J Lab Clin Med, 99; 46-55, 1982.

Hegarty V, et al, "Tea drinking and bone mineral density in older women", Am. J Clinical Nutrition, 71, 1003-1007, 2000.

Hernandez-Avila M, et al, "Caffeine, moderate alcohol intake, and risk of fractures of the hip and forearm in middle aged women", Am J Clin Nutr 54; 157-163, 1991.

Holick MF. Calcium and Vitamin D. Diagnostics and Therapeutics. Clin Lab Med. Sep;20(3):569-90, 2000.

Hollingbery PW, "Effect of dietary caffeine and aspirin on urinary calcium and hydroxiproline excretion in pre and postmenopausal women", Fed Proc, 44; 1149, 1985.

Jasminka I-E Brownbill RA, et al, Critical Factors for Bone Health in Women Across the Age Span: How Important Is Muscle Mass? Medscape General Medicine 4(2), 2002.

Johnell O, et al, "Bone morphology in epileptics", Calcified Tissue International, 28 (2), 93-97, 1979.

Kaneki M, Hedges SJ, Hosoi T, et. al. Japanese fermented soybean food as the major determinant of the large geographic difference in circulating levels of vitamin K2: possible implications for hip-fracture risk", Nutrition Apr;17(4):315-21, 2001.

Karasek M, Reiter RJ, "Melatonin and Aging", Neuronendocrinol Lett., 23 (suppl 1), 14-16, 2002.

Kleijnen J, Knipschild P, ter Riet G. Clinical trials of homoeopathy. Brit Med J 1991;302:316-23.

Lawoyin S, "Bone mineral content in patients with calcium urolithiasis" Metabolism, 28, 1250-1254, 1979.

Lambing CL. Osteoporosis 2003. Program and abstracts of the American Academy of Family Physicians 2003 Annual Scientific Assembly; October 1-5, 2003; New Orleans, Louisiana. Abstract 181.

Langer RD. Postmenopausal hormone therapy: the state-of-the-art 2003. Program and abstracts of the American Academy of Family Physicians 2003 Annual Scientific Assembly; October 1-5, 2003; New Orleans, Louisiana. Abstract 567.

Lanyon L.E, "Skeletal responses to physical loading, In G. Mundy & J.T.Martin (eds.), Physiology & Pharmacology of Bone, Vol. 107, 485-505. Berlin, Springer-Verlag, 1993.

Lees B, et al, "Differences in proximal femur bone density over two centuries", Lancet, 341, 673-675, 1993.

Linde, Clausius N, Ramirez G, et. al. Are the clinical effects of homeopathy placebo effects? A meta-analysis of placebo-controlled trials. Lancet 1997; 350:834-43.

Luborsky LB, et al, "Comparative Studies of Psychotherapies: Is it true that everybody has won and all must have prices?", Archives of General Psychiatry, 32, 995-1008, 1975.

Manson JE, Hsia J, Johnson KC, et al. Estrogen plus progestin and the risk of coronary heart disease. N Engl J Med. 2003;249:523-534.

McDougall J, "McDouggall's Medicine", New Century Publications, Piscataway, NJ, pg 67, 1985.

McLaren AM et al., "Urinary excretion of pyridinium crosslinks of collagen in patients with osteoporosis and the effects of bone fracture", Ann Rheum Dis 1992;51:648-51.

Mercola J, "Weekly e-healthy News", www.mercola.com, last accessed July 2004.

Michelson D, et al, "Bone mineral density in women with depression", New England Journal of Medicine, 335 (16) 1176-1181.

Murray T., Bone Health, www.doctormurray.com

National Osteoporosis Foundation: "Physician's Guide to Prevention and Treatment of Osteoporosis". Available at: http://www.nof.org/physguide/ inside_cover.htm Accessed December 30, 2003.

Neer RM, Arnaud CD, Zanchetta AR, et al. Effect of parathyroid hormone (1-34) on fractures and bone mineral density in post menopausal women with osteoporosis, N Engl J of Med, 2001, 344 (19) 1934-41.

Pennington J, "Bowes and Church's food Value of Portions Commonly Used", 17th Ed, Lippincott Williams and Wilkins, Philadelphia, 1998.

Pirello C, "Everything You Always Wanted to Know About Whole Foods But Were Afraid to Ask", Penguin, New York, 2004.

Prior J, et al, "Spinal bone loss and ovulatory disturbances", New England Journal of Medicine, 323 (18), 1221-1227, 1990.

Prochaska JO, Norcross JC, "Systems of Psychotherapy: A Transtheoretical Analysis", 3rd Ed., Pacific Grove, California, Brooks/Cole, 1994.

Prochaska JO, Norcross JC, Diclemente CC, "Changing for Good: A Revolucionary Six-Stage Program for Overcoming Bad Habits and Moving Your Life Positively Forward", Harper and Collins, NY 1994.

Quincannon Stanchich J, "Our protein choices", Christina's Living Healthy Journal, Vol. 6, No.1, pg. 1, 2004.

Reaven GM, "Syndrome X: Overcoming the silent killer that can give you a heart attack", New York, Simon & Schuster, 2000.

Recker R, "The Effect of Milk Supplements on Calcium Metabolism, Bone Metabolism, and Calcium Balance", American Journal of Clinical Nutrition, 41 (1985) 254.

Reilly D.T.et al,1986: "Is Homeopathy A Placebo Response?" The Lancet, Oct.18, 881-885.

Reiter R, "The aging pineal gland and its physiological consequences", Bioessays, 14, 169-175, 1992.

Rigotti NA, "Osteoporosis in women with anorexia nervosa", New England of Medicine, 311 (25), 1601-1605, 1984.

Rey, L. (2003). Thermoluminescence of ultra-high dilutions of lithium chloride and sodium chloride. Physica A: Statistical mechanics and its applications. 323, 67-74.

Robbins J, "The Food Revolution", Conari Press, Berkeley, CA, 2001.

Rozencwaig R, Grad BR, Ochoa J, "The role of melatonin and serotonin in aging", Med Hypotheses, 23: 337-352, 1987.

Rossouw JE, Anderson GL, Prentice RL, et al. Writing Group for the Women's Health Initiative Investigators. Risks and benefits of estrogen plus progestin in healthy postmenopausal women: principal results from the Women's Health Initiative randomized controlled trial. JAMA. 2002;288:321-333.

Sandyk R, Anastasiadis PG, Anninos PA, Tsagas N. "Is postmenopausal osteoporosis related to pineal gland functions?", International Journal of Neuroscience, 1992;62:215-225.

Schulz M.L, "Awakening Intuition: using your mind-body network for insight and healing", Three Rivers Press, New York, 1998.

Schurgers LJ, Vermeer C. Determination of phylloquinone and menaquinones in food. Effect of food matrix on circulating vitamin K concentrations. Haemostasis. 2000 Nov-Dec;30(6):298-307

Scofield A.M.: Experimental Research in Homeopathy-A Critical Review," The British Homeopathic Journal, Vol.73, Nos.3 and 4, July and Oct, 1984, Pags.161-180 and 211-226.

Sellmeyer DE, Stone KL, Sebastian A, et al. "A High Ratio of Dietary Animal to Vegetable Protein Increases the Rate of Bone Loss and the Risk of Fracture in Postmenopausal Women", *Am J Clin Nutr.* 2001;73:118-122

Shearer, "Role of vitamin K and Gla proteins in the pathophysiology of osteoporosis and vascular calcification". MJ.Curr Opin Clin Nutr Metab Care 2000 Nov;3(6):433-8

Spencer H, et al, "Alcohol-Osteoporosis", Am J Clin Nutr 41; 847, 1985.

Uebelhart D et al. "Urinary excretion of pyridinium crosslinks: a new marker of bone resorption in metabolic bone disease", Bone Miner 1990; 8:87-96.

University of California San Francisco, The Wellness letter, July 2002.

Van Meurs, J B.J. Ph.D., Rosalie A.M. Dhonukshe-Rutten, M.Sc., et al, "Homocysteine Levels and the Risk of Osteoporotic Fracture, The New England Journal of Medicine May 13, 2004;350:2033-2041

Weaver C.M, et al, "Absorbability of Calcium from Common Beans", Journal of Food Science, 58 (1993) 1401-3.

Weaver C.M, et al, "Dietary Calcium: Adequacy of a Vegetarian Diet", American Journal of Clinical Nutrition, 59 (Sup) 1994: 1238S-41S.

Colbin, Annemarie. Food and Our Bones. New York: Plume, a division of The Penguin Group, 1998

Conrad, Chris. Hemp: Lifeline to the Future. Novato, CA: Creative Xpressions Publications, 1994

Erasmus, Udo. Fats that Heal, Fats that Kill. Burnaby, Canada: Alive Books, 1993

Kushi, Michio. How to See Your Health: Book of Oriental Diagnosis. New York: Japan Publications, Inc., 1980

Lu, Henry C. Chinese Natural Cures. New York: Black Dog & Leventhal, Inc., 1994

Ohsawa, Georges. You Are All Sanpaku. New York: Citadel, 1965

Ohsawa, Georges. Zen Macrobiotics. Los Angeles, CA: Ohsawa Foundation, Inc., 1965

Rose, Richard. The HempNut Health and Cookbook. Santa Rosa, CA: Book Publishing Co, Summertown, TN, 2004

Veith, Ilza. The Yellow Emperors Classic of Internal Medicine. Berkeley, CA: University of California Press, 1949

Waters, Alice. Chez Panisse Vegetables. New York, NY: Harper Collins, 1996

Weil, M.D., Andrew. Eating Well for Optimum Health. New York: Alfred A. Knopf, 2000

Recipe Index